EVERYDAY HEALTH HACKS

Quick Fixes to Prevent
Disease and Improve
Your Well-Being

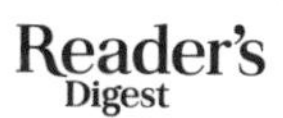

A READER'S DIGEST BOOK

ISBN 978-1-62145-513-4
eBook ISBN 978-1-62145-514-1

Portions of this book were previously published in *Stealth Health: How To Sneak Age-defying, Disease-fighting Habits Into Your Life Without Really Trying.*

We are committed to both the quality of our products and the service we provide to our customers. We value your comments, so please feel free to contact us.

Reader's Digest Adult Trade Publishing
44 South Broadway
White Plains, NY 10601

For more Reader's Digest products and information, visit our website:
www.rd.com (in the United States)
www.readersdigest.ca (in Canada)

Printed in the United States

10 9 8 7 6 5 4 3 2 1

NOTES TO OUR READERS
The information in this book should not be substituted for, or used to alter, medical therapy without your doctor's advice. For a specific health problem, consult your physician for guidance.

Reader's Digest publishes the advice of expert authorities in many fields. But the use of a book is not a substitute for legal, accounting, or other professional services. Consult a competent professional for answers to your specific questions. This publication is sold with the understanding that the contributors and the publisher are not engaged in rendering legal advice. Laws vary from state to state, and readers with specific issues should seek the services of an attorney.

Products or active ingredients, treatments, and the names of organizations that appear in this publication are included for informational purposes only; the inclusion of commercial products in the book does not imply endorsement by Reader's Digest, nor does the omission of any product or active ingredient or treatment advice indicate disapproval by Reader's Digest. When using any commercial product, readers should read and follow all label directions carefully. The publisher and the contributors specifically disclaim any responsibility for any liability, loss, or risk (personal, financial, or otherwise) that may be claimed or incurred as a consequence, directly or indirectly, of the use and/or application of any of the contents of this publication.

CONTENTS

EVERYDAY HEALTH HACKS

DAWN TO DUSK

1 **Wake up with the sun.** Sleep with your window coverings halfway open. That way, the natural light of the rising sun will send a signal to your brain to slow its production of melatonin and increase its production of adrenaline, a signal that it's time to wake up. When the alarm goes off, you'll already be half awake. Even better: go to bed early enough so that waking up when the sun shines through your window still gives you the recommended seven hours of shut-eye.

2 **Get your blood flowing.** Before you open your eyes, lift your arm and stretch each finger, then your hand, wrist, and arm. Next, move on to the other arm, then your toes, feet, ankles, and legs. End with a neck and back stretch that propels

you out of the bed. You've just limbered up your muscles and joints, and enhanced the flow of blood throughout your body, providing an extra shot of oxygen to all your tissues.

3 **Take your daily vitamin.** They are called vital amino acids for a reason. Keep a bottle of multivitamins on the kitchen counter right by the coffeemaker so you remember to take one every morning.

4 **Simplify your morning routine.** For truly relaxing mornings, reduce the number of choices and decisions you make to the bare minimum. Make your morning decisions the night before: what clothes to wear, what breakfast to eat, what route to take to work, and so on.

5 **Allow the scent of caffeine to jump-start your day.** By using a programmable coffeemaker, you can wake to the smell of coffee. Buy the absolute best coffee you can afford (fresh beans are preferred). The scent of strong coffee will pull you out of bed like few other motivations.

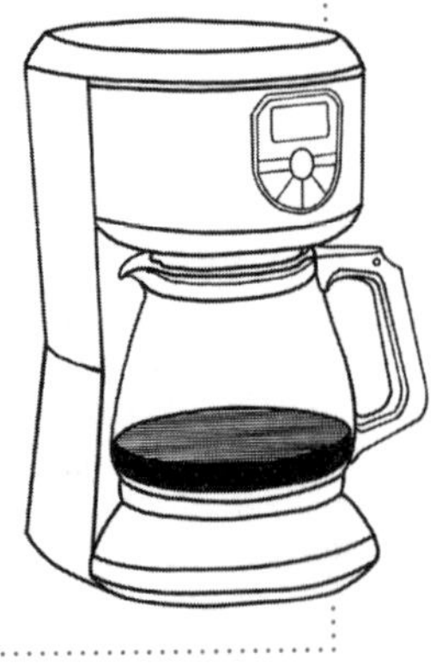

6 **Brush or scrape your tongue.** There's no better way to rid yourself of morning breath and begin your day minty-fresh and clean. After all, more than three hundred types of bacteria take up residence in your mouth every night. Brushing your teeth is not enough.

7 **Let yourself be a sweetie.** Use real sugar in your coffee or drink a cup of orange juice. University of Virginia researchers tested the memories of healthy sixty- to eighty-year-olds and found that those who had a small amount of sugar in the morning even before breakfast had better memory recall that day on into the following day. We're talking small amounts, however—about a teaspoon or less. (So put down that doughnut.)

8 **Strengthen your bones for the day ahead.** Swallowing 500 milligrams (mg) of a calcium supplement, either calcium citrate or calcium carbonate, will deter loss of bone tissue as you age. Each has its pluses and minuses, but calcium citrate is easier for your body to absorb. The recommended daily intake is 1,000 mg, so depending on how much you're getting from your foods, you may need another 500 mg before you go to bed.

9 **Rehydrate, rehydrate, rehydrate.** You've been fasting all night, and you wake each morning dehydrated. By drinking 8 ounces of water, you can rapidly rehydrate.

10 **Make your morning active.** Studies find that as little as thirty minutes of walking, yoga, weight lifting, or other workouts in the morning will produce endorphins that last most of the day. People doing morning workouts are more likely to stick with their exercise regimen because they get it out of the way and don't have all day to come up with diversions and excuses.

11 **Don't forget bye-bye kisses.** Kiss or hug all your loved ones in your house before you leave. Having this brief physical connection with those you love (including pets) soothes stress and provides you with a positive start to your day, as well as keeps you focused on what's really important.

12 **Limit your starting routine to fifteen minutes.** Don't spend much time getting coffee, settling in, reading emails, or checking messages. You are at your freshest and most productive at the beginning of the day. A prolonged morning routine removes your positive edge and makes your afternoon more stressful. Jump into the important work quickly and read the nonessential emails after you've accomplished some more important tasks.

13 **Assess your day's emotional challenges.** Think of this as a "be mentally prepared for" list. Inventory the tough phone calls, boring meetings, challenging customers, frustrating red tape, infuriating rush-hour drives, droning detail work, and other mental challenges you are likely to face. Then accept that they are inevitable, and prepare yourself to get through them without anger, frustration, or impatience. It's usually not our work that gets us down—we all should enjoy our work!—but rather the challenges that lie along the periphery of the job.

14 **Schedule some social time.** You probably work with people you like and with whom you have developed work relationships. Each morning should have a short period of social time with colleagues to build camaraderie. Make it at an appropriate time, and don't let a day go by without doing it.

15 **Set an hourly alarm.** This will be your signal throughout the day to take a break, get up and stretch, walk around the building, and so on.

16 **Listen to your mother and sit up straight.** Our tendency to slump while we're typing or sitting can cause fatigue, carpal tunnel syndrome, and back pain. Every time your alarm beeps or your phone rings, consider it a reminder to straighten your spine, pull back your shoulders, and lift up your neck.

17 **Loosen your tie (if you're wearing one).** Researchers have found that tighter ties increase eye pressure, a risk factor for glaucoma.

18 **Start your day with a cup of hot cocoa.** Research finds that one cup of cocoa a day for five days can increase blood flow in the brain, hands, and legs and helps regulate blood pressure. Choose a brand that isn't loaded with sugar or hydrogenated oil, such as Ghirardelli.

19 **Enjoy the latest audiobook or learn a new language while you drive.** You can borrow audiobooks from the library or download them from various subscription services on the Internet. Even bumper-to-bumper traffic is less stressful when you're in the thick of an interesting story.

20 **Practice good automobile ergonomics.** Don't just buckle up. Before you leave, make sure your headrest is set directly behind your head, aligned with the top of your ears. Adjust your seat and steering wheel for maximum comfort. Check each mirror to make sure you don't need to lean or crane your neck for best vision.

21 **Do some "traffic-light yoga."** Lift your legs and stretch them for thirty seconds. This reduces the risk of blood clots from sitting too long in one position. Put one arm behind your neck and stretch it by holding on to the elbow with the opposite arm, then switch sides. Do one of these stretches every time traffic comes to a halt.

22 **Work in short bursts.** The downside to multitasking is that it is difficult to sustain creativity or intensity for long stretches. Our brains work in cycles of creativity. Try working for an hour or so, get up for five minutes to stretch, walk around, or do some calisthenics. This will also help you from sitting for too long at your desk, which has been shown to be unhealthful.

23 **Give yourself daily kudos.** Take time to praise yourself for doing things well. When you've completed a task, tell yourself—out loud—what a good job you've done. You'll get a psychic burst of energy and confidence that will help you maintain your cool amid the workplace madness.

24 **Spread the praise around.** It's better to give than to receive. Provide praise and recognition to others at work whenever appropriate. You will feel good by making others feel good, and that feeling will tend to spread.

25 **Soothe your soul twice a day.** While reading poetry or religious writings, the cadence, words, and images will soothe your soul. If you're not into poetry or religion, try listening to a few of your favorite songs.

26 **Take a break to slide down the wall.** Find a private place to lean against a wall, slide down to a squatting position, and stay there for a few minutes without looking down, just feeling your spine against the wall. Breathe deeply (in through your nose, out through your mouth) and focus on one peaceful thought. Press your feet into the floor as you hold this position and picture the stress oozing out of your body into the earth. When you stand up, shake out your arms and legs and return to work refreshed.

27 **Reserve thirty minutes at the end of your workday.** It may seem strange when starting your day, but this is your opportunity to transition from work to home. During this last half hour, you'll finish answering emails, update your to-do list for the next day, and clean off your desk.

28 **Go for an after-dinner walk.** After eating is a great time for a stroll through the neighborhood. Walking and digesting both burn calories. To make it interesting, play a game of learning two new things about your neighbors on each walk, either through observation or conversation. Playing this kind of game will make your walk go quicker and keep it more interesting. The best bonus is the health-promoting effects of the walk.

29 **Play a game with your partner or kids.** Try a board game, work on a puzzle, or play a game of cards. This will keep the television off and stimulate brain cells, and the social bonding with your loved ones contributes mightily to emotional and physical health. Try old-fashioned games like backgammon, dominoes, checkers, hearts, or chess. Crossword puzzles are great fun, as are visual, number, and logic puzzles that you can get online.

30 **Play with your pet for fifteen minutes.** Studies show significant stress reduction benefits from playing with pets, particularly those that can interact with you. Use a laser light to drive your cat slightly crazy (the laughing you'll do as you watch it chase the light will have its own health benefits). Teach your cat to fetch by tossing a crumpled piece of paper. Hide treats around the house and watch your dog go on his own treasure hunt.

31 **Do something totally mindless for thirty minutes.** Maybe watch the junkiest show you can find on TV, hold a computer solitaire tournament with yourself, soak in a steamy, scented bath, or just lie on the couch listening to a favorite piece of music and stare at the ceiling. The idea here is that your mind is disengaged, not focused on anything, and allowed to run free in a kind of "active meditation."

32 **Slowly sip a glass of really good wine.** If you're used to Two-Buck Chuck, then a $15 bottle of Merlot is just the ticket. If you're a moderate oenophile, you might reach for a $50 bottle of Bordeaux. The idea is that you savor this one glass. While you're identifying the fruits you taste and the elements in the bouquet, the wine will be providing significant heart-healthy antioxidants shown to reduce your risk of heart disease.

33 **Savor a piece of good quality dark chocolate.** Ounce for ounce, chocolate contains more healthy antioxidants, which repair damage to cells and prevent cholesterol from oxidizing (making it stickier), than any other antioxidant champs, including tea, blueberries, and grape juice. It's well known for its ability to soothe a troubled mind. It only takes a 1-ounce piece to provide the perfect post-dinner sweetness we often crave without a lot of fat or calories. Keep the chocolate dark—70–80 percent cocoa has the most antioxidants—and plain, without the extra sugar and calories from caramel, nougat, or other goodies.

34 **Dance for twenty minutes.** If jazz or cheek-to-cheek dancing are not your thing, play some high-energy rock music and pretend you're in a mosh pit. Either way, you'll get twenty minutes of physical activity and, if you're doing the mosh pit thing, you'll burn as many calories as if you were jogging. An added bonus: improved coordination and, if you do a lot of dips, some good stretches. Plus, this is a great way for younger parents to engage their kids in physical activity—the whole family can "bust a move" until just one is left standing.

READY FOR EVERY SEASON

1. **Wash your hands often.** Hand washing—the single best way to protect yourself in flu season—should last for at least twenty seconds (two rounds of "Happy Birthday"). Proper hand washing includes five steps: wet, lather, scrub, rinse, and dry. The water can be warm or cold, as long as it is clean. When lathering, make sure to soap up the back of your hands, between your fingers, and under your nails.

2. **Carry hand sanitizer with you.** Although washing with soap and water is the best way to wash your hands, sometimes that is not readily available. The next best option is to use an alcohol-based hand sanitizer that contains at least 60 percent alcohol.

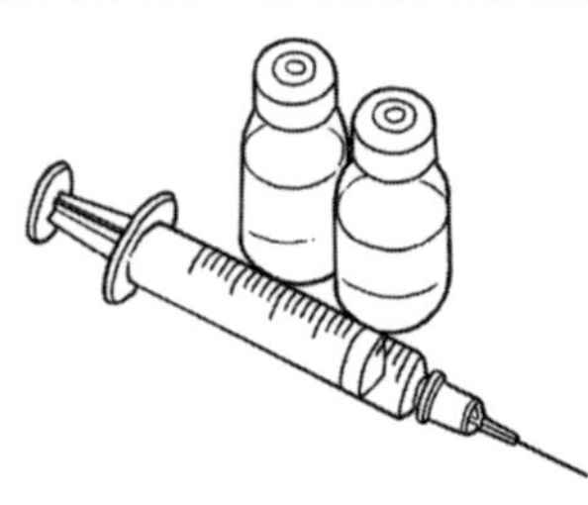

3 **Get a flu shot every fall.** The CDC recommends everyone (above the age of six months) get the flu shot every flu season. Kids between the ages of six months and eight years old may need two doses during the same season. Everyone above the age of eight only needs one dose.

4 **Talk to your doctor about the shingles vaccine.** The CDC recommends that healthy adults fifty and older get two doses of the shingles vaccine called Shingrix.

5 **Put a box of tissues wherever people sit.** Strategically place boxes of tissues around your house, your workplace, your car. Don't let aesthetics thwart you (find a cute tissue-box holder). You need tissues widely available so that anyone who must cough or sneeze or blow his or her nose will do so in the way least likely to spread germs.

6 **Sneeze and cough into your arm or tissue.** Whoever taught us to cover our mouths when we cough or sneeze was thinking in the right direction. But don't use your bare hand! That just puts the germs right on your hands, where you can spread them to objects and other people. Instead, hold the crook of your elbow over your mouth and nose when you sneeze or cough if a tissue isn't handy.

7 **Wipe your nose—don't blow.** Your cold won't hang around as long, according to a University of Virginia study. Turns out that the force of blowing not only sends the gunk out of your nose into a tissue but propels some *back* into your sinuses. If you need to blow, blow gently, and blow one nostril at a time.

8 **Keep your hands to yourself.** Remember the golden equation for getting sick: germ gets on hands, hands touch face, germ enters body, you get sick. So keep your hands in your pockets and to yourself. A note about gloves: wearing gloves can be tricky, as they can increase cross contamination.

9 **Change or wash your hand towels every three or four days.** When you wash them, use hot water in order to kill the germs.

10 **Sip a cup of goldenseal tea.** The herb, often found in over-the-counter remedies mixed with echinacea, may boost your immune system, preventing colds and other infections.

11 **Use your knuckle to rub your eyes.** It's less likely to be contaminated with viruses than your fingertip. This is particularly important given that the eye provides a perfect entry point for germs, and the average person rubs his eyes or nose or scratches his face twenty to fifty times a day.

12 **Microwave your toothbrush on high for ten seconds.** This will kill germs that can cause colds and other illnesses. You think it gets your teeth clean, and it does, but once you're done brushing, your toothbrush is a breeding ground for germs. Sterilize it in the microwave before you use it, store it in hydrogen peroxide (rinse well before using), or simply replace it every month when you change the page on your calendar and after you've had a cold.

13 **Buy a hygrometer to monitor your home's humidity.** You want your home to measure around 50 percent. A consistent measure higher than 60 percent means mold and mildew may start to set in your walls, fabrics, and kitchen. Lower than 40 percent and the dry air makes you more susceptible to germs. These can be found easily online or at many stores such as Target and Walmart. Pricing can range from $10 to $100, depending on how many special features you want.

14 **Don't pressure your doctor for antibiotics.** Colds and flu (along with most common infections) are caused by viruses, so antibiotics—designed to kill bacteria—are totally ineffective. They can hurt, however, by killing off the friendly bacteria that are part of our immune defenses. If you've used antibiotics lately, consider a course of probiotics, whether through supplements, yogurt or kefir, or fermented foods like raw sauerkraut. Your tummy will appreciate these replacement troops of friendly bacteria. And don't forget to feed these little guys with "prebiotics," healthy dietary fiber like onions, garlic, and greens.

15 **Try a garlic supplement every day.** People taking garlic—raw, cooked, or taken as a supplement—were not only less likely to get a cold, but if they did catch one, their symptoms were less intense and they recovered faster.

16 **Eat a container of yogurt every day.** People who ate one cup of yogurt—whether live culture or pasteurized—had 25 percent fewer colds than non-yogurt eaters. Start your yogurt eating in the summer to build up your immunity before cold and flu season starts. Keep it sugar free to avoid unwanted calories, adding your own fruit if you want.

17 **Leave the windows in your house open a crack in winter.** Not all of them, but one or two in the rooms in which you spend the most time. This is particularly important if you live in a newer home, where fresh circulating air has been the victim of energy efficiency. A bit of fresh air will do wonders for removing bacteria.

18 Lower the heat in your house five degrees.

Dry air in an overheated home provides the perfect environment for cold viruses to thrive. When your mucous membranes (nose, mouth, and tonsils) dry out, they can't trap those germs very well. Lowering the temperature and using a room humidifier helps maintain a healthier level of humidity in the winter.

19 Open your sinuses with some finger pressure.

Open your sinuses with some finger pressure. If you have clogged sinuses due to a cold or allergies, rub them with your index fingers (make sure to wash your hand thoroughly first). Start just above your brow line. Place your finger pads just above your nose, press down and rub outward, tracing your brow line as you go. Repeat two or three times. Then place the pads of your fingers below your eyes and to the sides of the bridge of your nose, rubbing outward and moving downward with each stroke. Use your thumbs to massage your cheekbones, making small circles starting at the center of your face and moving out toward your ears. Finally, place your thumbs on your temples and massage them in small circles.

20 **Start preparing three days before a trip.** Boosting your immune system with doses of echinacea and vitamin C can help prepare your body for travel. There are more germs on trains and planes than you can shake a stick at. Don't ruin your trip by getting sick.

21 **Protect against ticks.** When enjoying the outdoors, protect yourself against ticks. Wear clothing that covers your arms and legs. Make sure to tuck your pants into your socks (or use tape around any openings). Avoid walking through overgrown areas and wear light-colored clothing.

22 **Check for ticks.** When you get home, check your whole body. Use a fine-tooth comb to check your hair/scalp and check all folds of your skin. Get the mirror out to check for hard-to-see places, if you don't have someone to help.

23 **If you find a tick, don't panic.** Remove it as soon as possible, using a set of fine-tipped tweezers. Grab the tick as close to the skin's surface as possible and pull upward, with steady, even pressure. After removing the tick, make sure to clean the bit area thoroughly with rubbing alcohol or soap and water. If you develop a fever or rash within several weeks of the removal, see your doctor.

24 **Stay safe in the sun.** Make sure to have some sort of shade available when you are spending some time in the sun. But don't think you can skip the sunscreen if you are in the shade! Make sure you put on a broad-spectrum sunscreen with at least SPF 15 before you go outside.

25 **Apply a Vaseline shield.** If it's cold and windy, your face may suffer a case of windburn. A thin coating of Vaseline on exposed skin—particularly your cheeks, nose, chin, ears, and neck—will help prevent it. If you don't like petroleum products, try a natural alternative, like cocoa or shea butter, unrefined coconut oil, or even olive oil. Easy-to-find brands include Burt's Bees and Waxelene.

26 **Don't walk with your hands in your pockets.** If you slip, you want your hands free to help you regain your balance.

27 **Buy a pair of Yaktrax.** These amazing rubber and wire devices slip over the bottom of your boots and help prevent you from slipping on the ice. They are available at sporting goods stores and on the Internet.

28 **Remember snow's first cousin: ice.** So wear rubber-soled boots with good traction, go slowly, don't carry too many packages, and give yourself extra travel time to get wherever you're going, whether that's on foot or by car.

29 **Look for signs of frostbite.** Patches of white or pale gray, waxy-textured skin are signs of frostbite. Get indoors and get immediate medical attention.

30 **Use rubber dishwashing gloves over woolen gloves.** It may look silly but will keep your gloves dry whether you're shoveling snow or making snowballs.

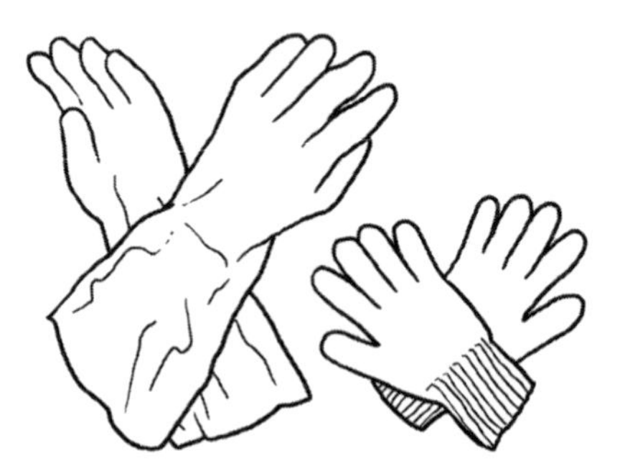

31 **Make sure your boots aren't too tight.**

If they're too small or you've stuffed them with too many pairs of bulky socks, you won't have enough blood circulating to your feet and they'll get even colder. Wool or polypropylene socks are a good choice.

32 **Protect your eyes and skin.**

Smear on some sunscreen and lip balm if you're out in the snow on sunny days. And slip on a pair of sunglasses or goggles to protect your eyes from the snow's glare. A sunny day in winter is often brighter and more dangerous to your eyes than the same sun in summer, thanks to the reflection off ice and snow.

33 **Dress in layers.**

Make your first layer a shirt or long underwear made of synthetic microfibers, such as polypropylene. These wick sweat away from the body so you don't get too chilled. Avoid cotton, which gets wet and stays wet. Put on a fleece top over your first layer and then a windproof jacket.

34 **Equip your car for driving in snowy conditions.** Clean snow off the car before you start driving, make sure your windshield wipers work well, clean off your headlights, and use snow tires or chains if you need them. Stock your trunk with a shovel, tow rope, ground sheet (for fitting chains), rubber gloves, plastic ice scraper, blanket, and flashlight.

35 **Launch a preventive blitz at the very first hint of a cold.** These measures either reduce the length of time you suffer with a cold or help prevent a full-blown cold from occurring. Suck on a zinc lozenge until it melts away, every two waking hours, or use a zinc-based nasal spray such as Zicam. Take one 250-milligram capsule of the herb astragalus twice a day until you are better. Cook up a pot of chicken soup. Roast garlic in the oven (drizzle a whole clove with olive oil, wrap in aluminum foil or parchment paper, and roast for an hour at 400°F), then spread the soft garlic on toast and eat.

BREATHING EASIER

1 **Breathe like a singer.** Breathe from your belly for at least five minutes every day. This kind of breathing, called diaphragmatic breathing, involves training and strengthening your diaphragm so it requires less effort to take each breath. To do it, inhale deeply through your nose, filling your lungs from the bottom up. If you are doing it right, your stomach will pooch out. Exhale and repeat.

2 **Enforce a no-smoke zone in your house.** Secondhand smoke can damage your lungs just as much as the smoke from your own cigarette.

3 **Breathe in through your nose.** In hot, dry, or very cold weather, or in dusty/polluted air, breathe in through your nose and out through your mouth. Our nasal passages are designed to filter the air and regulate its temperature and humidity. If you breathe in through your mouth, everything—dust, coldness, and so on—goes straight into the lungs.

4 **Eat one kiwifruit every morning.** They're rich in vitamin C, which acts as a natural antihistamine.

5 **Keep your thermostat set above 65°F in the winter.** If you set it too low, you're encouraging the growing of mold in damp air. The heat dries out the air, preventing mold growth. Of course, too-dry air can also irritate your lungs and sinuses. The perfect humidity in a home is around 50 percent.

6 **Put a shelf by the front door for shoes.** Encourage your family and guests to remove their shoes before entering to reduce the amount of dust, mold, and other allergens tracked in.

7 **Climb stairs.** The kind of exercise that makes your heart beat faster, like climbing stairs, riding a bike, or walking briskly, is very important for keeping your heart and lungs in good shape. For instance, studies find that walking about fifteen minutes at a time, three to four times a day, improved breathing in people with emphysema, a lung disease.

8 **Pop a fish oil supplement every morning.** Most airway problems, including asthma, are related to inflammation. Omega-3 fatty acids, which are the main ingredient in fish-oil supplements, reduce inflammation.

9 **Expand your chest like a cocky rooster.** To help expand and boost your lung capacity, lie on the floor with your knees bent and your feet flat on the floor. Place your hands behind your head and bring your elbows together so they're nearly touching. As you inhale, slowly let your elbows drop to the sides so your arms are flat on the floor when your lungs are full. As you exhale, raise your elbows again.

10 **Work in ten to twenty crunches a day.** Your abdominal and chest muscles allow you to suck air in and out. Strengthen them.

11 **Find ways to eat more tomatoes.** Try making spaghetti sauce or tomato and basil salads. British researchers found that people who ate tomatoes three to four times a week had improved lung function and experienced less wheeziness and fewer asthma-like symptoms.

12 **Wear a face mask.** Wearing a face mask when working around toxic dust or fumes is a must. Even simple household tasks like sanding paint could send damaging fragments into your lungs, says Kevin Copper, a Virginia Commonwealth University Medial Center pulmonologist. And wearing a mask when you are sick or when there is a flu or other airborne illness outbreak not only helps keep you safe but can prevent you from spreading the disease to others. The face mask should fit snugly but comfortably, include multiple layers of fabric, allow you to breathe without restriction, and be able to be laundered and machine dried without damage.

13 **Turn on the AC.** Air conditioners remove mold-friendly moisture and filter allergens entering the house. Just make sure to clean or change the filters often, or you'll make things worse.

14 **Plant flowers.** The pollen in flowers rarely causes allergies, due to its large size. It's the microscopic pollens from many bushes and trees that are culprits for people with allergies.

15 **Change your home air filter.** Once a season should do the trick. You'll not only breathe easier but increase energy efficiency and extend the life of your HVAC unit.

MATTERS OF THE HEART

1. **Take a B vitamin complex every morning.** When Swiss researchers asked more than two hundred men and women to take either a combination of three B vitamins (folic acid, vitamin B6, and vitamin B12) or a placebo after they had surgery to open their arteries, they found that levels of homocysteine, a substance linked to an increased risk of heart disease, were 40 percent lower in those who took the vitamins. The placebo group had no change. Plus, the vitamin group had wider-open blood vessels than those taking the sugar pill.

2. **Go to bed an hour earlier tonight.** A Harvard study of seventy-thousand women found that those who got less than seven hours of sleep had

a slightly higher risk of heart disease. Researchers suspect lack of sleep increases stress hormones, raises blood pressure, and affects blood sugar levels. Keep your overall sleeping time to no more than nine hours, though, because the same study found women sleeping nine or more hours had a slightly *increased* risk of heart disease.

3 **Eat fish.** Have it grilled, sautéed, baked, or roasted—just have it. Women who ate fish at least once a week were one-third less likely to have a heart attack or die of heart disease than those who ate fish only once a month. The benefits are similar for men. Regular fish consumption reduced the risk of atrial fibrillation—rapid, irregular heartbeat—a major cause of sudden death.

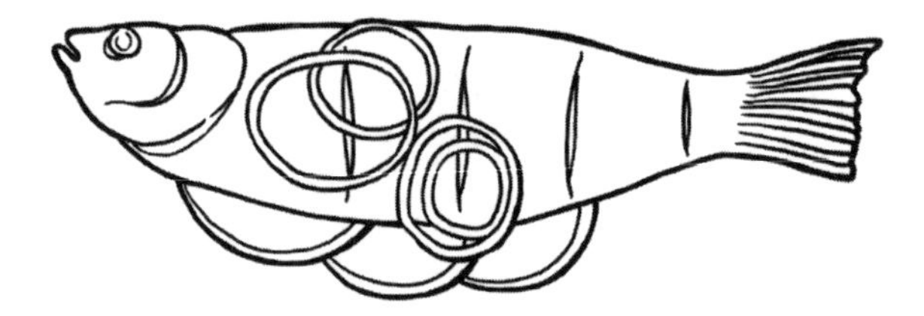

4 **Eat a high-fiber breakfast cereal at least four times a week.** Women who ate 23 grams of fiber a day—mostly from cereal—were 23 percent less likely to have heart attacks than those who consumed only 11 grams of fiber. In men, a high-fiber diet slashed the chances of a heart attack by 36 percent.

5 **Make fresh salad dressing with one tablespoon of flaxseed oil.** It packs a whopping 7 grams of omega-3 fatty acids, which are a great way to improve your overall heart health.

6 **Drink at least two cups of tea a day.** Black or green, it doesn't seem to matter. That's the result of a Dutch study that found only 2.4 percent of five thousand healthy Rotterdam residents who drank two or more cups of tea a day had a heart attack within six years, compared with 4.1 percent of those who never drank tea. Another major analysis of seventeen studies on tea drinkers found three cups a day could slash the risk of a heart attack by 11 percent.

7 **Stir a handful of hazelnuts into a vegetable-and-chicken stir-fry.** Just one and a half ounces of these healthful nuts a day can reduce your risk of cardiovascular disease. Also try crushing them and use to coat fish or chicken, then bake.

8 **Include beans or peas in four of your dishes every week.** People who followed this advice slashed their risk of heart disease by 22 percent compared to those who ate fewer legumes. Aim for one cup per day. You'll be getting at least 300 micrograms (mcg) of folate. People who consumed at least that much folate slashed their risk of stroke 20 percent and their risk of heart disease 13 percent more than those who got less than 136 mcg per day of the B vitamin. If you don't like beans, try an orange (55 mcg), spinach (58 mcg per cup raw spinach), romaine lettuce (62 mcg per cup), or tomatoes (27 mcg per cup). Since January 1998, wheat flour has been fortified with folic acid, the synthetic form of folate, adding an estimated 100 mcg per day to the average diet.

9 **Take a baby aspirin every day.** The tiny tablet slashes the risk of heart disease by nearly a third in people who have never had a heart attack or stroke but who were at increased risk because they smoked, were overweight, had high blood pressure, or some other risk factor. Double-check with your doctor that there's no reason for you *not* to take aspirin daily.

10 **Eat cherries every day.** Studies find the anthocyanins (plant chemicals) that give cherries their scarlet color also work to lower levels of uric acid, a marker for heart attacks and stroke. When cherries are out of season, try sprinkling dried cherries on your salad or substituting a cup of cherry juice for orange juice in the morning.

11 **Drink an 8-ounce glass of water every two hours.** Women who drank more than five glasses of water a day were half as likely to die from a heart attack as those who drank less than two. This is likely due to the fact that maintaining good hydration keeps blood flowing well. Dehydration can cause sluggish blood flow and increase the risk of clots forming. Water works best when it comes to improving blood flow; soda is worthless.

12 **Cook with ginger or turmeric twice a week.** They have anti-inflammatory benefits, and inflammation is a major contributor to heart disease.

13 **Go to the bathroom whenever you feel the urge.** A full bladder causes your heart to beat faster and puts added stress on coronary arteries, triggering them to contract, which could lead to a heart attack in people who are vulnerable.

14 **Drive with the windows closed and the air-conditioning on.** This reduces your exposure to airborne pollutants, which reduces something called "heart rate variability," or the ability of your heart to respond to various activities and stresses. Reduced heart rate variability, also called HRV, has been associated with increased deaths among heart attack survivors as well as the general population.

15 **Call a friend and arrange dinner.** Having a very close relationship with another person, whether it's a friend, lover, or relative, can halve the risk of a heart attack in someone who has already had one.

16 **Pay attention to the basics.** Nearly everyone who dies of heart disease, including heart attacks, had at least one or more of the conventional risk factors: smoking, diabetes, high blood pressure, or high cholesterol levels. You can find dozens of tips on lowering your blood pressure, reducing your cholesterol, stabilizing your blood sugar, and quitting smoking online.

17 **Treat untreated depression.** If you find you're having trouble getting out of bed in the morning, have lost interest in your normal activities, or just feel really blah, call your doctor. You may be depressed, and untreated depression significantly increases your risk for a heart attack.

18 **Adopt a dog.** The power of furry friends to improve heart health is proven. Not only will a dog force you to be more active (think about all the extra walking you'll be doing), but the companionship and unconditional affection a pooch provides has been shown to reduce the risk of heart attack and other cardiovascular problems.

19 **Use soy milk for a healthy heart.** Packed with potent phytoestrogens, soy has been credited with protecting your heart and promoting stronger bones. Make sure that it's fortified with calcium; otherwise, you're missing a great opportunity to achieve some bone-building. Allergic to soy? Almond milk, rice milk, flax milk, coconut milk, and hemp milk all have great health-supporting properties. Of course, get the no-sugar-added versions for best results.

20 **Sprinkle ground flaxseeds for heart health.** Use just one teaspoon over your cereal, yogurt, smoothie, or eggs. Next to fish and organic eggs, flaxseeds are one of the best sources of omega-3 fatty acids.

21 **Record yourself while you sleep.** If you hear yourself snoring (or if your partner has been kicking you a lot), make an appointment with your doctor. You may have sleep apnea, a condition in which your breathing stops hundreds of times throughout the night. It can lead to high blood pressure and other medical problems, and even increase your risk for heart attack and stroke.

22 **Eat six or more small meals a day.** People who ate six or more times a day had significantly lower cholesterol than those who ate twice a day, even though the "grazers" got more calories and fat. The differences in cholesterol between the two groups were large enough to reduce the grazers' risk of coronary heart disease 10–20 percent. Just make sure those six meals are truly small.

23 **Make all your sandwiches with whole grain bread.** Cutting back on simple carbs like white bread and eating more complex carbs, like whole grain bread and brown rice, can increase HDL levels slightly and significantly lower triglycerides, another type of blood fat that contributes to heart disease.

24 **Use paper filters when brewing your coffee and skip the espresso.** Two substances found in brewed coffee, kahweol and cafestol, increase cholesterol levels. But paper filters trap these compounds, so they're only a problem if you drink espresso or use coffeemakers without filters.

25 **Use olive oil in your homemade salad dressing.** Diets rich in the kind of monounsaturated fat found in olive oil reduced

LDL cholesterol in people with diabetes or metabolic syndrome—a cluster of risk factors including low HDL, high insulin levels, and obesity—just as well as following a low-fat diet. Other sources of monounsaturated fats are avocados, tree nuts, and canola oil.

26 **Add half a tablespoon of cinnamon to your coffee beans.** Before starting the pot, add cinnamon to the grounds. Six grams of cinnamon per day (about half a tablespoon) reduced LDL cholesterol in people with type 2 diabetes nearly 30 percent and cut total cholesterol 26 percent.

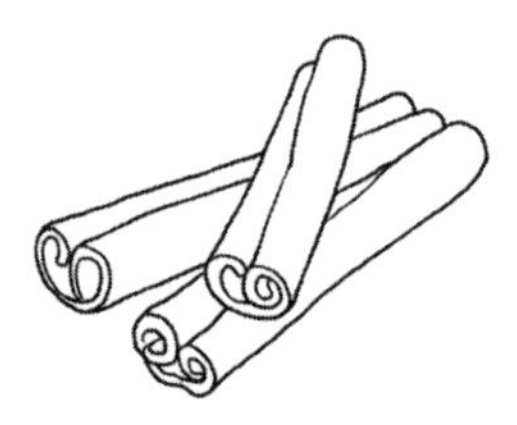

27 **Have a few glasses of cranberry juice every day.** Cut it with seltzer or water so you get less sugar. Or get the unsweetened kind. Cranberries are a rich source of anthocyanins, flavonols, and proanthocyanidins, plant chemicals that prevent LDL cholesterol from oxidizing, a process that makes it more likely to stick to artery walls, and they also keep red blood cells from getting too sticky. They also initiate a complex chemical reaction that helps blood vessels relax. Plus (the part you were waiting for) they decrease LDL cholesterol levels, and three glasses of cranberry juice a day can raise HDL levels up to 10 percent.

28 **Eat a grapefruit every other day.** Grapefruits are particularly high in pectin, a soluble fiber that can help reduce cholesterol levels. Grapefruits interfere with the absorption of several medications, however, so check with your doctor first. Other good sources of pectin include apples and berries.

29 **Use honey in your tea instead of sugar, and instead of jam on PB&J sandwiches.** Total and LDL cholesterol levels dropped in healthy people after they drank a solution containing honey, but not after they drank solutions containing glucose or artificial honey. After fifteen days of the honey drink, participants' HDL levels rose and homocysteine levels dropped. Homocysteine is an amino acid linked to an increased risk of heart disease, stroke, and peripheral vascular disease (reduced blood flow to the hands and feet).

30 **Enjoy a glass of wine every evening with dinner.** Studies find a daily glass of wine can boost levels of HDL cholesterol. If you don't drink, there's no reason to start. But if you enjoy wine, make it a red one—red wines are three to ten times higher in plant compounds called saponins believed to be responsible for much of wine's beneficial effects on cholesterol.

31 **Pop edamame as a snack.** Just half a cup contains nearly 4 grams of fiber, not to mention the soy isoflavones in these soybeans. Consumption of both has been linked to lower cholesterol. Edamame is now available in the frozen food section of the supermarket.

32 **Whip up a batch of guacamole.** Several studies find that eating one avocado a day as part of a healthy diet can lower your LDL as much as 17 percent while raising your HDL.

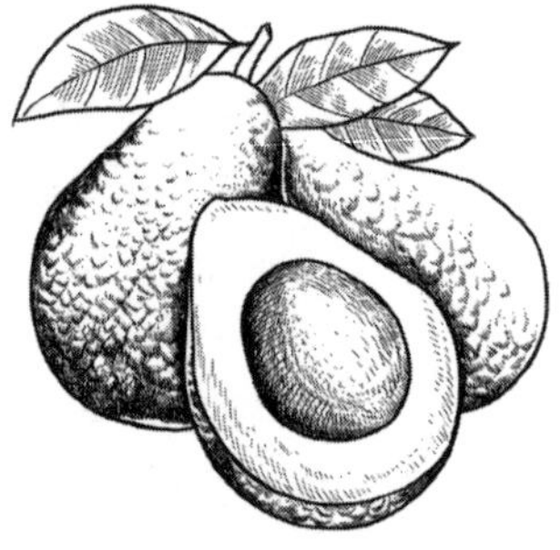

33 **Spend ten minutes a day doing strength-training exercises.** You don't have to do these at a gym—push-ups, squats, leg lifts, and hip extensions all count. And they count when it comes time to count your cholesterol levels. Strength training lowered total cholesterol 10 percent and LDL cholesterol 14 percent among women who worked out for forty-five to fifty minutes three times a week. If you can't manage that amount, start with ten minutes a day, six days a week, and gradually work up.

34 **Have a glass of purple grape juice every day.** Rich in cholesterol-lowering flavonoids, grape juice is the perfect drink, particularly if you don't like red wine.

35 **Have oatmeal for breakfast every morning.** There's a reason oat manufacturers are allowed to boast about the grain's cholesterol-lowering benefits: plenty of research has proved them. Rich in soluble fiber called beta glucan, oatmeal can drop your LDL 12–24 percent if you eat one and a half cups regularly. Choose quick-cooking or old-fashioned oats over instant.

STOP DIABETES BEFORE IT STARTS

1 **Don't skip a meal.** First off, your blood sugar drops like a rock when you're starving (hence the headache and shakiness). Second, when you do eat, you flood your system with glucose, forcing your pancreas to release more insulin and creating a dangerous cycle.

2 **Add at least one day of resistance training.** You'll build more muscle than you will by walking, and the more muscle mass you have, the more efficiently your body burns glucose and the less hangs around in your blood.

3 **Add a cup of decaffeinated coffee if you simply must have that doughnut.** British researchers found that combining decaf with

* The tips in this chapter apply to Type 2 diabetes. Type 1, sometimes called junvenile diabetes, cannot be prevented.

simple sugars (like those in doughnuts, cakes, and cookies) reduces the blood sugar spike the sweets create. Regular coffee does not have the same benefit. The reason? While plant chemicals in coffee slow the rate at which your intestines absorb sugar, caffeine delays sugar's arrival in muscles, keeping it in the bloodstream longer.

4 **Drink a cup of skim milk and eat 8 ounces of nonfat unsweetened yogurt a day.** A study of three thousand people found that those who were overweight but ate a lot of dairy foods were 70 percent less likely to develop insulin resistance (a precursor to diabetes) than those who didn't. Turns out lactose, protein, and the fat in dairy products improves blood sugar by filling you up and slowing the conversion of food sugars to blood sugar.

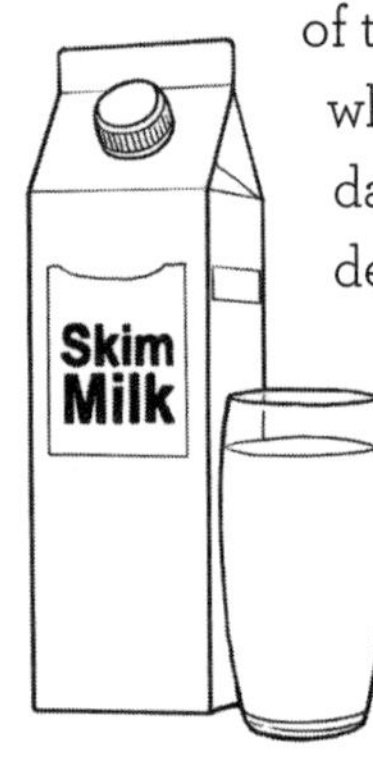

5 **Buy bread products that have at least 3 grams of fiber and 3 grams of protein per serving.** They'll slow absorption of glucose and decrease the possible insulin spikes, says J. J. Flizanes, a nutritionist and owner of Invisible

Fitness in Los Angeles. Plus, the hearty dose of fiber and protein will keep your stomach feeling satisfied longer.

6 **Serve up a spinach salad for dinner.** Spinach is high in magnesium, which a large study suggests can prevent the development of type 2 diabetes.

7 **Sprinkle cinnamon over your coffee, yogurt, cereal, and tea.** Researchers from Pakistan had volunteers with type 2 diabetes take either 1, 3, or 6 grams of cinnamon or a placebo for forty days. Those taking the fragrant spice saw their blood glucose levels drop by 18–29 percent, depending on how much cinnamon they took.

8 **Munch on baked chips.** Made without saturated fat found in fried foods, baked chips are an excellent substitute when you are craving something crunchy and salty. University of Minnesota scientists evaluated three thousand people and found those with the highest blood levels of saturated fats were twice as likely to develop diabetes.

9 **Watch a comedy after eating.** A Japanese study found that people with diabetes who laughed soon after eating (while watching a comedy) had significantly lower blood sugar levels than those who listened to a boring lecture. The connection held even for those without diabetes.

10 **Eat some now and some later.** Dish out your breakfast, lunch, and dinner, but then divide each meal in half. Eat half to start with, then the other half in a few hours. Eating several small meals rather than three large meals helps avoid the major influx of glucose that, in turn, results in blood sugar surge and a big release of insulin.

11 **Eat half a cup of beans a day.** These high-fiber foods take longer to digest, so they release their glucose more slowly. Studies find that just half a cup a day can help stabilize blood sugar and insulin levels.

12 **Lose weight.** Seven or eight pounds may make a large difference. It can significantly raise your motivation and energy levels, thus powering you toward more weight loss.

13 **Be physically active.** Aim for thirty minutes a day. Studies show that this can reduce your risk of diabetes by up to 25 percent.

14 **Add more fiber.** Eat more vegetables, fruits, whole grains, nuts, seeds, beans, and lentils on a regular basis. Together, hacks 12, 13, and 14 in this section can slash your risk of diabetes by nearly 60 percent.

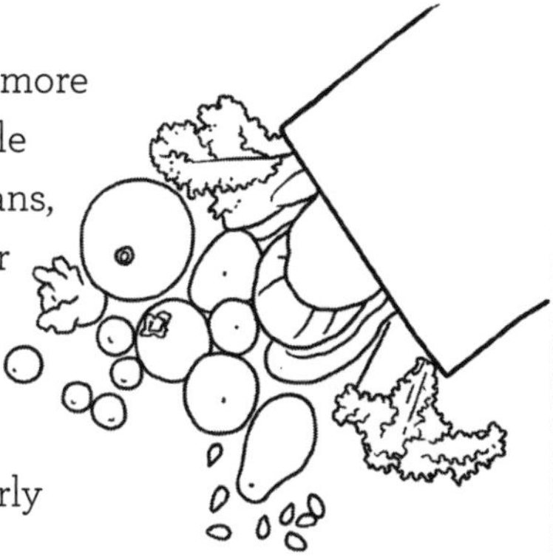

15 **Eat potatoes boiled with the skin on.** The effect of potatoes on blood sugar depends on how the potatoes are prepared. No need to unspud yourself completely! Also, new potatoes tend to have fewer simple carbs than the other types of potatoes. Another trick: cook the potatoes today and eat them tomorrow after a night in the fridge. Studies show that even if you reheat them, they'll have far more resistant starch, which functions like fiber and lessens the blood sugar response.

16 **Lighten your glycemic load.** A food's glycemic index measures how much a food will increase your blood sugar after eating it. Foods with low glycemic load—like beans, bran cereal, brown rice, whole wheat bread, and nuts—have less impact on your blood sugar than foods with a high glycemic load—like white rice, spaghetti, potatoes, cornflakes, and sugary juices and drinks. Eating more low-glycemic-load foods will help you keep your blood sugar steady and avoid the light-headedness and "shakes" associated with blood sugar drops, which usually follow spikes.

17 **Sprinkle powdered psyllium seed over your salad, yogurt, and scrambled eggs.** The powdered form is easier to mix into foods, like meat loaf or sauces. But the whole husks are fine too; both are inexpensive. Studies find the high-fiber seed may help lower elevated blood sugar.

KEEPING CANCER AWAY

1 **Serve sauerkraut at your next picnic.** A Finnish study found that the fermentation process involved in making sauerkraut produces several other cancer-fighting compounds including ITCs, indoles, and sulforaphane. To get all the probiotic benefits, get the raw fermented type, as opposed to the canned, which is pasteurized and has no beneficial bacteria. To reduce the sodium content, rinse the sauerkraut before eating.

2 **Eat your fill of broccoli.** But steam it rather than microwaving it. Broccoli is a cancer-preventing superfood, one you should eat frequently. But take note: a Spanish study found that microwaving broccoli destroys 97 percent of the vegetable's cancer-protective flavonoids. So steam it, eat it raw, or add it to soups and salads. And broccoli is a great source of protein.

3 **Snack on Brazil nuts.** These easy-to-find, large, three-sided Amazon tree nuts are a rich form of selenium, a trace mineral that convinces cancer cells to commit suicide and helps cells repair their DNA. A Harvard study of more than a thousand men with prostate cancer found those with the highest blood levels of selenium were 48 percent less likely to develop advanced disease over thirteen years than men with the lowest levels. And a dramatic five-year study conducted at Cornell University and the University of Arizona showed that 200 micrograms of selenium daily—the amount in just two Brazil nuts—resulted in 63 percent fewer prostate tumors, 58 percent fewer colorectal cancers, 46 percent fewer lung malignancies, and a 39 percent overall decrease in cancer deaths.

4 **Pop a calcium supplement with vitamin D.** A study out of Dartmouth Medical School suggests that the supplements reduce colon polyps (a risk

factor for colon cancer) in people susceptible to the growths.

5 **Add garlic to everything you eat.** Garlic contains sulfur compounds that many say stimulate the immune system's natural defenses against cancer and may have the potential to reduce tumor growth. Studies suggest that garlic can reduce the incidence of cancer by as much as a factor of twelve!

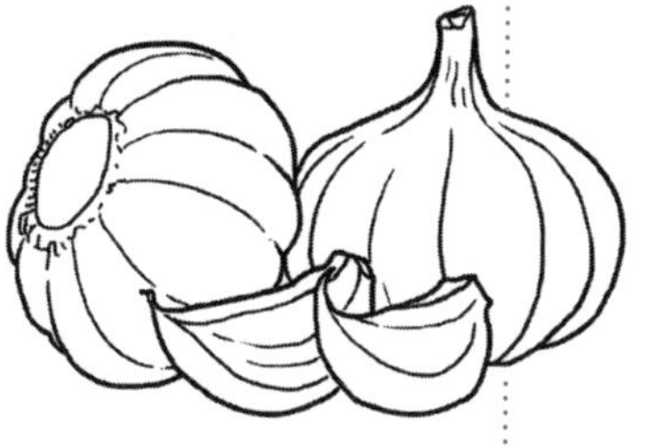

6 **Make tomato sauce.** Sauté two cloves of crushed garlic in two tablespoons of olive oil, then mix in a can of low-sodium diced tomatoes. Stir gently until heated and serve over whole wheat pasta. The lycopene in the tomatoes protects against colon, prostate, and bladder cancers; the olive oil helps your body absorb the lycopene; and the fiber-filled pasta reduces your risk of colon cancer.

7 **Add a cantaloupe to your diet.** Eat a few pieces every morning. Cantaloupe is a great source of carotenoids, plant chemicals shown to significantly reduce the risk of lung cancer.

8 Put some lemon slices in your water pitcher.

Not only will it make your water taste fresher but citrus fruits and juices—eaten fresh, juiced, or used in marinades and the like—may cut the risk of mouth, throat, and stomach cancers by half, Australian researchers found.

9 Have your partner feed you grapes.

They're great sources of resveratrol, the cancer-protecting compound found in wine, but don't have the alcohol of wine, which can increase the risk of breast cancer in women. Plus, the closeness such an activity engenders (we hope) strengthens your immune system.

10 Limit exposure to the sun to fifteen minutes.

Too little vitamin D may increase your risk of multiple cancers. The best source is exposure to UVB rays found in natural and artificial sunlight. But too much sun can increase your risk for cancers of the skin.

11 **Don't smoke.** Cigarette smoking causes about 80 to 90 percent of lung cancer deaths in the United States. The most important thing you can do to prevent lung cancer is to not start smoking, or to quit if you smoke.

12 **Keep a healthy weight.** Research has shown that being overweight or obese raises a person's risk of getting some cancers, including endometrial (uterine), breast in postmenopausal women, and colorectal cancers.

13 **Get tested for hepatitis C.** Hepatitis is inflammation of the liver, which is most often caused by a virus. In the United States, the most common type of viral hepatitis is hepatitis C. Over time, chronic hepatitis C can lead to serious liver problems including liver damage, cirrhosis, liver failure, or liver cancer.

14 **Try some black tea.** Black and green tea are jammed with heart-healthy antioxidants that provide more than just an energy-boosting punch. In addition to contributing to healthier arteries, they may also help prevent cancer.

15 **Sprinkle scallions over your salad.** A diet high in onions may reduce the risk of prostate cancer by as much as 50 percent. But the effects are strongest when they are eaten raw or lightly cooked. Try scallions, Vidalia onions, shallots, or chives for a milder taste.

BOOSTING YOUR BONES

1. **Add almonds to everything.** They're packed with bone-strengthening calcium. Just 1 ounce, about a handful, provides 70 mg of calcium.

2. **Drink one cup of tea a day.** That's all it took in a study of 1,256 women ages sixty-five to seventy-six to increase their bone density by 5 percent. That translates to a 10–20 percent reduction in fracture risk! Another study found that among

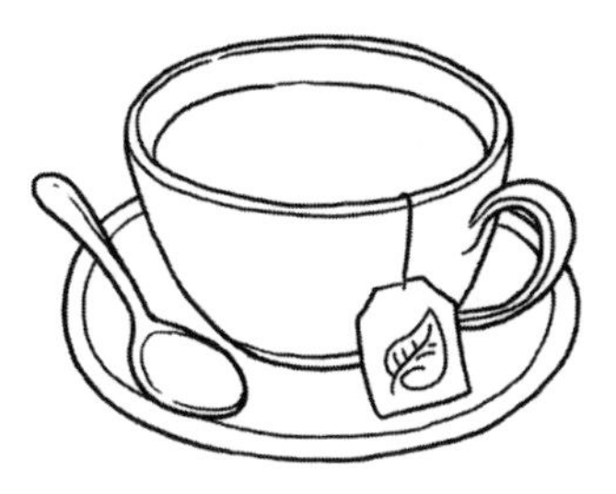

more than one thousand Chinese men and women, those who regularly drank tea (usually green tea) had denser bones than those who didn't.

3 **Make two glasses of water a day mineral water.** Mineral water contains calcium, and a study published in *Osteoporosis International* in 2000 found that your body absorbs the mineral just as well from water as it does from milk. Make sure the water is labeled "mineral water," not "spring water."

4 **Do twelve to sixteen squats each day.** Squats are particularly beneficial for your hips, which are especially prone to fracture.

5 **Jump around for ten minutes every day.** Jump rope, do jumping jacks, jump on a minitrampoline (or a big one). Just jump. It's one of the best all-around exercises for building bone.

6 **Try some coleslaw or stuffed cabbage rolls for dinner once a week.** Cabbage is rich in vitamin K, a vitamin that helps turn on a bone-building protein called osteocalcin.

7 **Take the right kind of calcium at the right time.** Calcium citrate, for instance, is absorbed more easily on an empty stomach, so take it before meals. Calcium carbonate, the cheapest and most common type of supplement, is absorbed best when taken with food, particularly acidic foods such as citrus juice or fruit.

8 **Sign up for tai chi.** Several studies found tai chi cut the risk of falling nearly in half and cut the rate of fractures even in people who had falls, notes Joseph Lane, chief of the metabolic bone disease service at the Hospital for Special Surgery in New York City. Ideally, you should practice tai chi for ten to fifteen minutes at a time, once or twice a week, to gain the benefit.

9 **Choose brown rice over white rice.** It's got three times the calcium. Brown rice hasn't been processed and still has its high-fiber nutrients.

10 **Get your calcium in unexpected places.** Look for calcium-fortified orange juice, cereals, and frozen yogurt. Sardines and canned salmon, as well as some dark green leafy vegetables (think kale and collard greens), are also great sources.

11 **Add nonfat powered milk to soups, casseroles, baked goods, and drinks.** It's an easy, unobtrusive way to sneak more calcium into your diet, particularly if you don't like drinking milk.

12 **Add hand weights to your daily exercises.** Weight-bearing exercise is critical for starving off bone loss. Take them on your daily walk, use them while waiting for your tea to be ready or while listening to a commercial break during your true-crime podcast.

13 **Learn to cook with yogurt.** Many cultures, particularly Indian, use yogurt every day in cooking.

SAY YES TO SEX

1. **Have sex tonight!** Having intercourse regularly helps keep your sex drive in high gear by increasing the production of testosterone, which is the hormone mainly for libido in both men and women.

2. **Spend tonight planning a steamy vacation.** Even if you don't go, spending time together picturing where you'd go, looking at locations online, and imagining yourself in some tropical paradise will be enough for a libido booster to get you to bed—early.

3 **Make pesto and serve it over pasta.** Pesto contains pine nuts, great sources of arginine, the precursor for nitric oxide, a main ingredient in drugs like Viagra. Arginine helps open blood vessels, so blood flow improves.

4 **Initiate intimate contact.** Put your arms around your partner's waist and begin kissing the back of his/her neck. Hopefully, this will lead to something more. In addition to the obvious benefits of sex, you'll also be raising your heart rate, sending immune-boosting endorphins to your brain, and extending your life. Sexually active men live longer than those who had less lovemaking, and this most likely applies to women too.

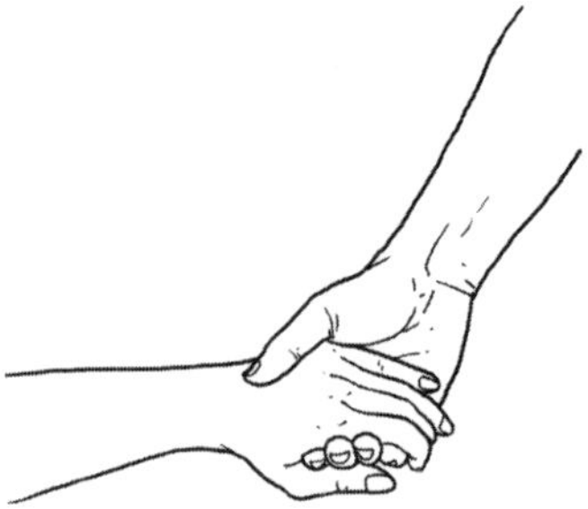

5 **Every time you pass your partner, reach out and touch/kiss him or her.** Don't allow these moments to go beyond the kiss or hug. Simply increasing the amount of physical contact you have with your partner will help with desire.

6 **Use protection with a new partner.** Condoms aren't just to prevent pregnancy; they can also protect you from sexually transmitted infections.

7 **Talk to your partner.** Knowing your partner's sexual history is important.

8 **Get tested.** Besides talking to your partner, the best way to protect yourself (and him or her) is to get tested on a regular basis. Some symptoms of sexually transmitted infections can be mistaken for other health issues, including age-related health problems.

9 **Practice Kegel exercises.** You know what Kegels are—they are the squeezing exercises your doctor told you to do after pregnancy or because you were having a bit of a problem with leaking urine. What the doctor may not have told you is that they are also great for strengthening the pubococcygeus muscle, essential for orgasm. To do Kegels, take a note of the muscle you use to stop urinary flow, then practice contracting

that muscle, gradually releasing it. Work up to twenty contractions three times a day. And Kegels aren't just for women. Men can also use them to strengthen their pelvic floor muscles as well.

SLEEP SWEETER AND DEEPER

1 **Create a transition routine.** This is something you do every night before bed, and it should be consistent to the point that you do it without even thinking about it. It can be as simple as turning out the lights, turning down the heat, washing your face, and brushing your teeth. Or it could be a series of yoga or meditation exercises. As you begin to move into your "nightly routine," your mind will get the signal that it's time to chill out and tune down, dialing down stress hormones and physiologically preparing you for sleep.

2 **Listen to your body.** Some experts believe sleepiness comes in cycles. If you get really sleepy at 10:00 p.m. and you push past it, you likely won't be able to fall asleep very easily for a while. If

you've noticed these kinds of rhythms in your own body clock, use them to your advantage. When sleepiness comes, get to bed; otherwise it might be a long time until you are ready to fall asleep again.

3 **Use lavender water to promote relaxation.** Put lavender water in a perfume atomizer and spray above your sheets and pillowcases before climbing in.

4 **Put your phone on Do Not Disturb mode.** Better yet, keep it away from your bed. You will be less tempted to check your phone in the middle of the night if you have to get out of bed to look at it.

5 **Choose the right pillow.** Neck pillows, which resemble a rectangle with a depression in the middle, can actually enhance the quality of your sleep as well as reduce neck pain. The ideal neck pillow should be soft, not too high, provide neck support, and be allergy tested and washable. A pillow with two supporting cores received good ratings while water-filled pillows provided the best night's sleep when compared to participants' usual pillows or a roll pillow. A pillow filled with a special "cool" material composed of sodium sulfate and ceramic fiber provided a much better night's sleep than one filled with polyester, because the cooler pillow kept the subjects' head cooler.

6 **Use thicker curtains or get blackout shades.** Even the barely noticeable ambient light from streetlights, a full moon, or your neighbor's house can interfere with the circadian rhythm changes you need to fall asleep.

7 **Keep your room tidy.** Clutter in your bedroom can distract from a good night's sleep. Smooth, clean surfaces act as a balm to your brain, helping to clear your worries and mental to-do lists.

8 **Move your bed away from any outside walls.** This will reduce noise, which could be a significant factor in insomnia. If the noise is still bothering you, try a white noise machine or turn on a floor fan.

9 **Warm your feet to cool your core.** The science is a little complicated, but warm feet help your body's internal temperature get to the optimal level for sleep. You sleep best when your core temperature drops. By warming your feet, you increase blood flow to your legs, allowing your trunk to cool.

10 **Sleep alone.** One of the greatest disruptors of sleep is the loved one next to you who might be snoring, kicking, or crying out (this includes pets). Eighty-six percent of women surveyed said their husbands snored, and half had their sleep interrupted by it. Men have it a bit easier; 57 percent said their wives snored, while 15 percent found their sleep bothered by it.

11 **Try to stop your snoring!** Consider these antisnoring tips: quit smoking, have a light meal for dinner and nix any alcohol, try Breathe Right strips, and make an appointment at a sleep center.

12 **Try a combination supplement before bed.** By taking 600 mg calcium and 300 mg magnesium before bed, not only will you be providing your bones with a healthy dose of minerals, but magnesium is a natural sedative. Calcium helps regulate muscle movements. Too little of either can lead to leg cramps, and even a slight deficiency of magnesium can leave you lying there with a racing mind.

13 **Have some melatonin and tryptophan.** A banana is a great natural source of melatonin, the sleep hormone, as well as tryptophan. The time-honored tradition, of course, is warm milk, also a good source of tryptophan. A handful of walnuts is a good source of tryptophan, an amino acid known to enhance sleep. Melatonin supplements—powders, pills, drops, and even gummies—are readily available.

14 **Drink water before bed, not fruit juice.** It can take an extra twenty to thirty minutes to fall asleep after drinking a cup of fruit juice, most likely because of the high sugar content in juice.

15 **Listen to an audiobook while you fall asleep.** Just as a bedtime story soothed and relaxed us as children, a calming audiobook can have the same effect with adults. Try poetry or a biography; stay away from horror novels. Or try a podcast!

16 **Simmer three or four large lettuce leaves in a cup of water.** After fifteen minutes, remove from the heat, add two sprigs of mint for flavor, and sip just before you go to bed. Lettuce contains a sleep-inducing substance called lactucarium, which affects the brain similarly to opium without the addictive side effects.

17 **Give yourself a massage.** Slowly move the tips of your fingers around your eyes in a slow, circular motion. After a minute, move down to your mouth, then to your neck and the back of your head. Continue down your body until you find you're so relaxed you're ready to drop off to sleep. You could also alternate massage nights with your significant other.

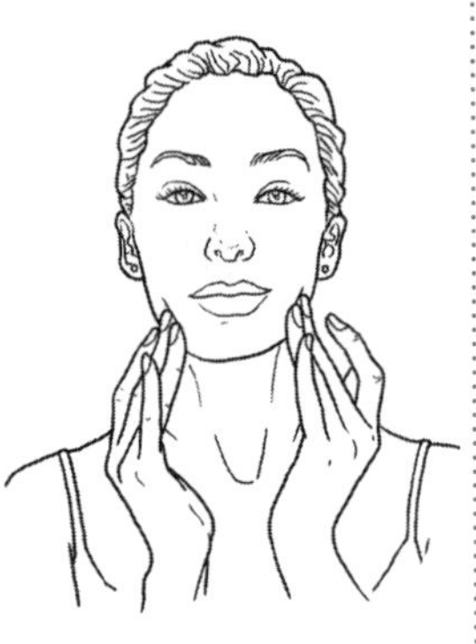

18 **Take a hot bath 90 to 120 minutes before bedtime.** Women with insomnia who took a hot bath during this window of time (water temperature approximately 105°F) slept much better that night. The bath increased their core body temperature, which then abruptly dropped once they got out of the bath, readying them for sleep.

19 **Use eucalyptus for a muscle rub.** The strongly scented herb provides a soothing feeling and relaxing scent. You can find eucalyptus oil to mix into a carrier oil or use a eucalyptus-scented cream.

20 **Tuck yourself in and spend ten minutes journaling.** This "data dump" will help turn off the repeating tape of our day that often occupies our minds, keeping us from falling asleep.

21 **Keep a notepad at your bedside along with a gentle night-light and pen.** If you wake in the middle of the night and you think of something important, you can quickly write it down, returning to sleep knowing you "caught" those thoughts. Alternatively, record the note on your smartphone.

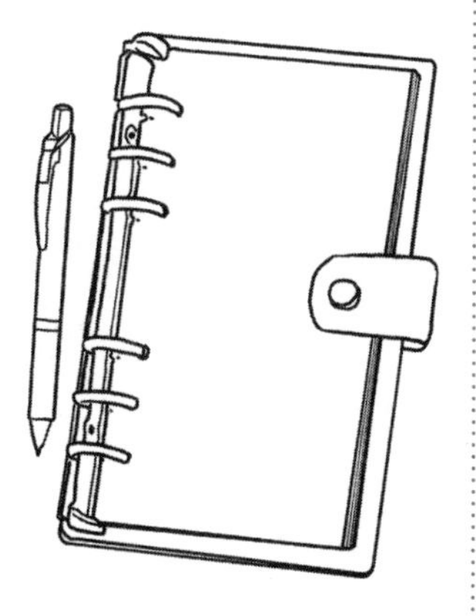

22 **Wake up at the same time each day.** Your whole day builds upon the time that you awake. This is what sets your body in motion into your daily activities. Consistency in your wake-up time allows your body to better know what to expect and to follow a comfortable daily rhythm. As the day goes by, your sleep drive will gradually build and maximize at the right point—not too early, not too late. We've all experienced how falling asleep too early or too late for one night can throw us off for days. Having a consistent wake-up time based on your unique schedule is crucial if you're having difficulties falling or staying asleep.

Use your bed for sleeping only. Don't do work on it, eat on it, or watch movies and TV while in it. Not only is that more hygienic, but you'll find it easier to fall asleep that way.

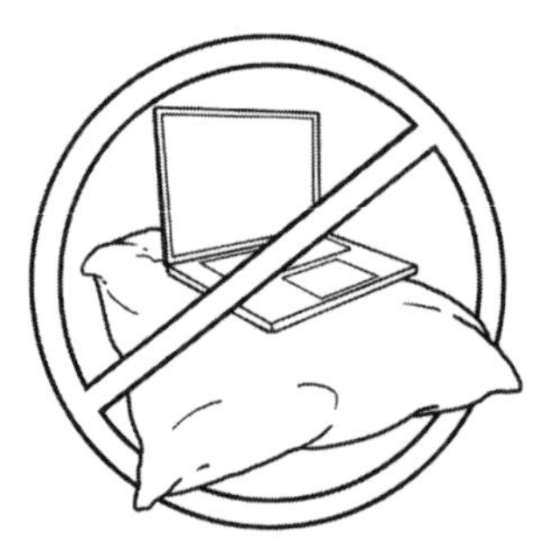

24 Roll out of bed, get clothes, shoes, and get exercising!

If you exercise first thing in the morning, you have no excuse. Research shows that people who plan to exercise in the morning are more likely to fit in their workouts than people who plan to exercise later in the day. Exercising in the morning may offer a side benefit: you'll sleep better at night. People who exercised at least 225 minutes per week in the morning had an easier time falling asleep at night than those who completed the same amount of exercise in the evening.

25 Drink your wine early in the evening.

Alcohol can sometimes make you feel drowsy and may help you fall asleep, but the sleep you get won't be as restful. Your brain waves and circadian rhythm can get out of whack, and your REM sleep—considered the most restorative—is blocked. Don't drink for two to three hours before bedtime and wake up more refreshed.

26 **Keep it cool.** Bedroom temperatures of 60–70°F are optimal.

27 **Timing is everything.** Eating large meals too close to bedtime has been shown to negatively affect sleep patterns in men and women. It can cause indigestion, and the feeling of fullness makes it more difficult to fall asleep. Limit your bedtime eating to small snacks. Experiment with going without even those and see if you get a better night's sleep.

28 **Wind down by candlelight.** The blue light emitted by TVs, iPads, phones, and computers can interfere with the brain's ability to release melatonin. Turn off all these devices for thirty to sixty minutes before going to bed. Instead, read a

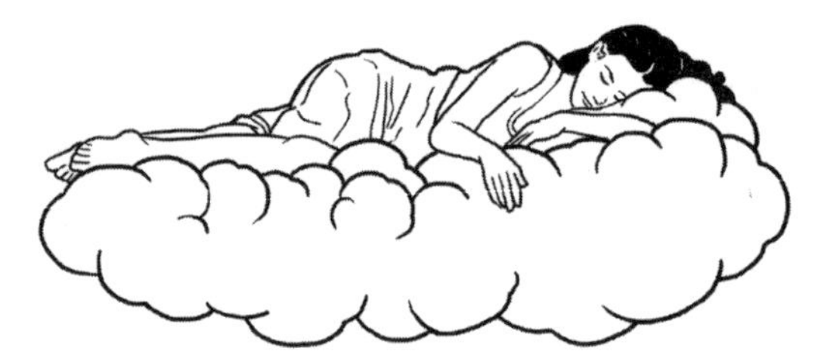

book, do a crossword, draw, or just sit quietly by a glowing candle.

29 **Go essential.** Oils, that is. These compounds extracted from plants are used in the practice of aromatherapy. Using aromatic oils can improve the health of the body, mind, and spirit. Lavender is the most popular oil, but rose, geranium, and sandalwood also enhance sleep. Some brands offer special sleep mixtures. Put several drops in your nighttime bath (hack 18) or rub a couple of drops in the palms of your hands and inhale. Diffusers also work well. Experiment to find the right scent for your bedtime routine.

GOOD-FOR-YOU GROCERIES

1 **First of all, buy fresh food!** The simplest, easiest, and plainest measure of the healthfulness of your food is whether it comes in boxes and cans or is fresh from the farm or fields. If more than half your groceries are prepared foods, then you need to evolve your cooking and eating habits back to the healthy side by picking up more fresh vegetables, fruits, seafood, juices, and dairy products.

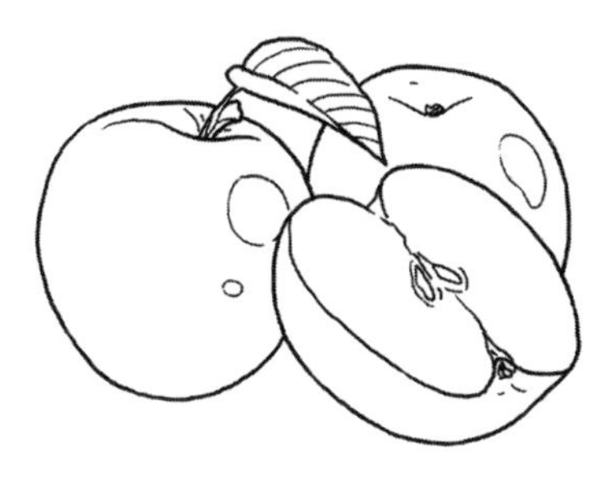

2 **Shop the perimeter of the store.** That's where all the fresh foods are. The less you find yourself in the central aisles of the grocery store, the more healthful your shopping trip will be. Peruse the perimeter of the store for the bulk of your groceries, then go into the aisles for staples that you know you need.

3 **Consider the departments, such as dairy, produce, and meat, as separate stores.** You wouldn't shop at every store during each trip to the mall so apply the same approach to the grocery store. Target the sections that are safe to browse through—the produce section, primarily—and steer clear of the dangerous sections such as candy, ice cream, and potato chips.

4 **Shop with a list.** Organize your shopping list based on the sections of the store. This will have you out of the supermarket quickly. By using a well-planned shopping list, you can resist the aisles of junk food, thereby saving your

home, family, and yourself from an overload of empty calories.

5 **Don't shop hungry.** Everyone has heard this one before, but it's worth repeating. Walking through the grocery store with your tummy growling can make you want to buy everything in sight. If you can't shop after a meal, be sure to eat an apple and drink a large glass of water before heading into the store.

6 **Buy a few days before ripe.** Buy fruit that's still a day or two behind ripeness. It will still be hard to the touch and bananas may be green, but it's wasteful if everything is overripe two days later. Feel carefully for bruises on apples, check expiration dates on bagged produce, and stay away from potatoes or onions that have started to sprout.

7 **Buy in season.** It's tempting to buy strawberries in December, but fresh fruit and vegetables are best when purchased in season, meaning they've come from relatively close to home. They often cost less, are tastier, and have less risk of pathogens such as E. coli.

8 **Look for organic whenever possible.** They may cost a few dollars more, but organically grown fruits and vegetables contain higher levels of cancer-fighting antioxidants than conventionally produced foods. If organic is too pricey for you, don't worry; organic or not, fruits and veggies are key to a healthy pantry.

9 **Try frozen.** Frozen fruits and vegetables are often flash frozen at the source, locking in nutrients. Stock your freezer with bags of frozen vegetables and fruits. You can toss the veggies into soups and stews, microwave them for a side dish with dinners, or thaw them at room temperature and dip them into low-fat salad dressing for snacks. Use the fruits for desserts, smoothies, and as ice cream and yogurt toppings.

10 **Stock up on canned tomato products.** A major exception to the "fresher is better" rule, canned tomato sauces and crushed and stewed tomatoes have higher amounts of the antioxidant lycopene than fresh, because they're concentrated. These are a godsend when it comes to quick dinners. And a great way to stock your pantry for emergencies.

11 **Eat beans.** Beans can be mixed with brown rice, added to soups and stews, pureed with onions and garlic into hummus for dipping, or served over pasta for a traditional pasta *e fagioli*. The hype about pasta raising blood sugar really comes down to what you are putting on your pasta. The soluble fiber in beans lowers blood sugar and insulin, making the combination of pasta and beans a healthful—as well as delicious—dish. Be sure to rinse them several times in the sink to get rid of excess sodium. And don't forget dried beans: they're cheaper and have no preservatives.

12 **Spend some time in the condiment aisle.** With the following basic ingredients you have the underpinnings for wonderful sauces, low-fat marinades, and low-salt flavorings: flavored ketchups and barbecue sauces (look for sugar-free varieties), horseradish, mustards, flavored vinegars, extra-virgin olive oil, capers, jarred olives, sun-dried tomatoes, Worcestershire sauce, hot pepper sauce, soy sauce, sesame oil, and teriyaki sauce.

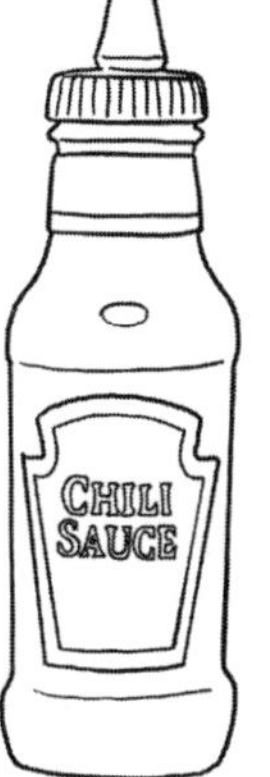

13 **Try the new whole grain alternatives.** There are wonderful whole grain pastas, couscous, and instant brown rice that cooks up in ten minutes instead of fifty, even whole grain crackers. While you're at it, pick up a bag of whole wheat flour to replace the white stuff in your canister.

14 **Look for prepared foods with the shortest ingredient lists.** The shorter the ingredient list, the healthier the food usually is. Of course, if the ingredients are sugar and butter, put the item back on the shelf.

15 **Beware of corn syrup.** It is a calorie-dense, nutritionally empty sweetener perhaps even worse than refined sugar and is reputed to be one of the main causes of America's obesity problem. A shocking number of foods and drinks are thick with it, including such apparently healthy foods as fruit juices, premade spaghetti sauces, and even bread. If a food has corn syrup in its first four ingredients, then it lacks the wholesomeness and healthiness you want.

16 **Be on the lookout for fiber.** You want at least 1 or 2 grams of fiber for every 100 calories you consume. An active woman needs 2,000 calories a day to maintain her weight, so get at least 20–40 grams of fiber every day.

17

Avoid partially hydrogenated oil and trans fats. They are hazards to your health and should be avoided. Common culprits include margarine and shortening, packaged snacks, ready-to-use dough, fried foods, and coffee creamers. Read food labels carefully, not just the marketing claims but the ingredients list.

18

Try dried shiitake mushrooms, which can be stored for years. They may look weird but toss them in some hot water for half an hour and you have a meaty, healthy addition to soups, stews, and sauces, not to mention a unique filling for tarts and omelets.

19

Rethink reaching for a package of ground meat. Go to the poultry section instead and pick up ground turkey, ground chicken, or soy crumbles. These work well for meatballs, meat loaf, or chili. This substitution can cut more than 30 percent of the calories and at least half of the fat and saturated fat in a 3-ounce serving.

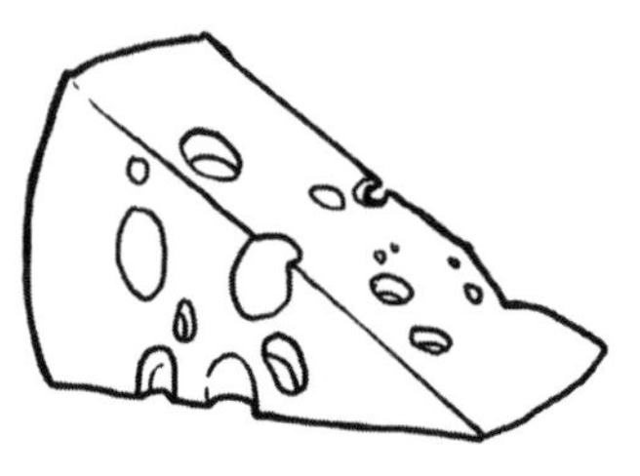

20 **Choose strong cheeses.** Instead of American, cheddar, or Swiss, pick up feta, fresh Parmigiano-Reggiano, or a soft goat cheese. You can use less of these strongly flavored cheeses and still satisfy your yen without damaging your waistline.

21 **Buy macadamia nut oil.** It has more healthful monounsaturated fats than any other oil in the world and a higher smoke point than olive oil, so there's no trans fatty acid formation when you cook. It makes any dish you make heart-healthier.

22 **Confirm that the wheat bread is whole wheat.** Some of the folks selling bread are trying to pull the wool (or is it wheat chaff?) over your eyes. Wheat bread is made from wheat, but if the first ingredient is refined wheat flour, then it's made from the same wheat as white bread—which means, stripped of fiber and nutrients, and in some cases, dyed brown for a fake healthy appearance. What you're really looking for are the words "whole wheat." That's the stuff with minimum refining and maximum beneficial nutrients.

23 **Buy plain yogurt and flavor it at home.** Pre-flavored yogurts have oodles of sugars that destroy any healthful benefits they once had. If you add a teaspoon of all-fruit jam at home, it'll still taste yummy, you'll consume far fewer useless calories, and you'll save lots of money.

24 **Buy healthy add-ins for plain cereals.** These include raisins, fresh berries, dried berries, almond slivers, pumpkin seeds, sesame sticks, and bananas. The best strategy is to buy unsweetened cereals, add your favorite flavors—which will allow you to bypass all the empty sugary calories—and you'll actually enjoy the cereal more. Keep a wide-mouth, well-sealed jar on your counter with

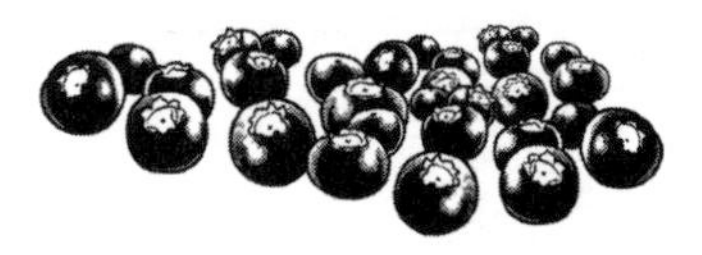

shelf-stable ingredients for quick access. Keep a scoop and ziplock bags handy, and you've got a nutritious meal or snack for home or on the go.

25 **Check juice labels.** Orange juice, although quite healthy, often has 20 grams of sugar in the average 8-ounce glass. Instead, try guava juice. It has three times more vitamin C and is loaded with potassium (a great blood pressure regulator) and beta-carotene.

26 **Look for hidden sources of sugar.** Cough syrups, chewing gum, mints, tomato sauce, baked beans, and lunch meats often contain sugar. Even some prescription medications contain sugar.

27 **Consider planting a garden.** Start with one vegetable or fruit. You will be more likely to eat it

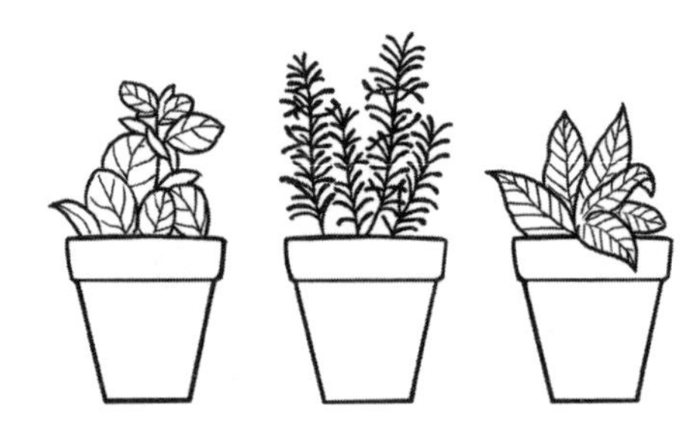

after spending time watching it grow and caring for it. Also try some herbs to use in place of salt for flavoring food.

28 **Go natural.** Stevia is a zero-calorie sugar substitute that comes in a variety of brands and forms, perfect for your morning coffee. Other great substitutes include erythritol and monk fruit sweeteners. They won't raise your blood sugar, and you can even use them in your favorite cookie recipe. You may never go back to cane sugar.

DELICIOUS AND NUTRITIOUS

1 **Serve raw vegetables at every meal.** Nearly everyone likes carrot sticks, celery sticks, cucumber slices, sugar snap peas, cherry tomatoes, and/or bell pepper strips. They're healthy, have virtually no calories, have a satisfying crunch, and can substantially cut your consumption of the more calorie-dense main course. So have a plate of raw vegetables in the center of the table, no matter what the meal is.

2 **Make a sandwich rule: more lettuce and tomato than meat.** The meat portion in the sandwich should be no higher than the thickness of a standard slice of bread. Pile on low-calorie slices of lettuce and tomatoes to the combined height of both slices of bread. Your sandwich tower has the height of the Empire State Building with the svelteness of the Eiffel Tower.

3 **Roast your vegetables.** These make great side dishes, are easy to make, delicious to eat, and amazingly healthful—plus they taste surprisingly sweet. They last well as leftovers, too, which means you can make large batches and serve throughout the week. Cut hearty root vegetables like parsnips, turnips, rutabagas, carrots, and onions into inch-thick chunks and arrange in a single layer on a cookie sheet. Drizzle with olive oil and sprinkle with kosher or sea salt, freshly ground pepper, and fresh or dried herbs. Roast in a 450°F oven until soft, about forty-five minutes, turning once.

4 **Use canned pumpkin for dessert.** Sprinkle it with cinnamon and mix in two packets of sweetener. Even if you eat the whole can, this dessert is only 140 calories and packs a healthy 9 grams of fiber. For a half cup you get 40 calories and 3.5 grams of fiber, not to mention tons of beta-carotene.

5 **Substitute cauliflower for carbs.** Add pureed cauliflower to mashed potatoes. You won't taste

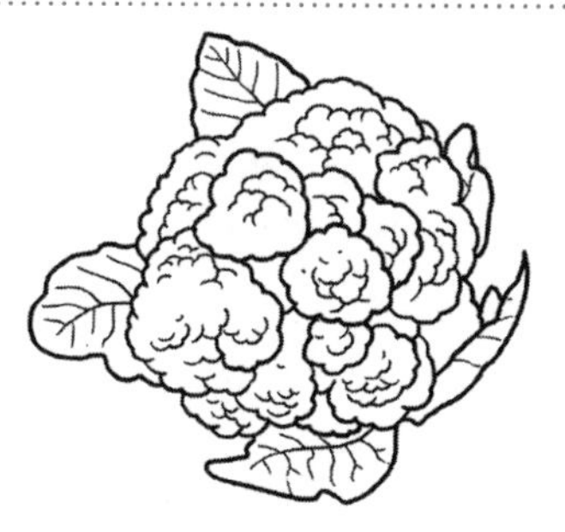

the difference, but you will get some extra fiber. Riced cauliflower can be used as a substitute for rice. Try pizza dough made from cauliflower.

6 **Have a beet salad for dinner.** These bright red veggies have virtually no fat, no cholesterol, no sodium, quite a bit of potassium, and 2 grams of fiber. Try roasting whole, peeled beets for forty-five minutes, chilling, then dicing into a summer salad.

7 **Add some flaxseeds, wheat germ, or other high-fiber option.** Mixed into the batter, they provide crunchiness to your cookies, muffins, and breads—and loads of fiber.

8 **Skip the movie theater popcorn.** Popcorn isn't a bad food. But it is a simple carb with little other nutritional value and, when bought at the theater, is often drowning in salt and fat. Better movie snacks are small bags of nuts or seeds and fresh or dried fruit. Just sneak them into the theater in your purse or a backpack.

9 **Mix up a sweet dessert.** Combine nonfat cream, unsweetened cocoa, a sugar substitute, and ice in a blender. Or mix mascarpone and the sugar substitute with whipped cream and a hint of lemon zest.

10 **Go half and half.** Mix half a regular soda with half a diet soda, half a carton of sweetened yogurt with half a carton of plain yogurt, or half a cup of regular juice with half a cup of seltzer. After two weeks, cut back to one-quarter sweetened to three-quarters unsweetened. Continue until you're drinking only the unsweetened version. Or try having a glass of iced water or soda water every *other* time you reach for a drink.

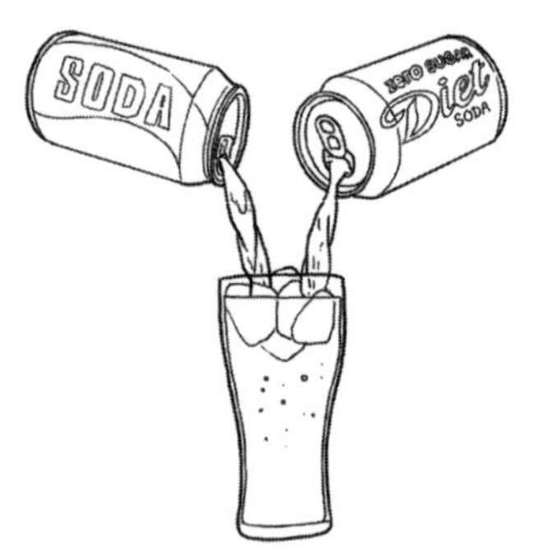

11 **Grant yourself a daily sugar "quota."** Use it on foods only where it matters most, like desserts. Don't waste it on dressings, spreads, breakfast cereals, and soda. This will reduce your daily sugar consumption and will help you lose your sweet tooth. Sugar is incredibly addictive: the more you eat, the more addictive it becomes and the more it takes to satisfy you. The opposite is also true: train your taste buds to become accustomed to less and you'll be satisfied with less.

12 **Avoid sports drinks.** They're loaded with sugar. Same with many protein powders.

13 **Choose low-fat products over regular.** The argument that low-fat versions don't taste as good just isn't true! Low-fat versions may not taste the way you are used to, but after a week or two of using the new version, you'll stop noticing the subtle difference in richness.

14 **Don't be taken in by the "other white meat" slogan.** Put simply, lean chicken is much less fatty than lean pork. A 3-ounce serving of broiled chicken breast (no skin) provides 140 calories, 27 from fat, and only one-third of that fat is saturated.

The same serving of roasted lean pork loin delivers 275 calories, 189 of them from fat, half of which is saturated. To top it off, the chicken has 6 grams more protein than the pork.

15 **Remove it if you can see it.** If there is fat on the meat or skin on the chicken, trim it off. If there is oil pooling on the top of the pizza, sop it up with a paper towel. If there is dressing pooled at the bottom of your salad, pour it off. If there's a pool of juice under a cooked steak (and it's not a sauce), drain it, and if there's fat at the top of a bowl of stew or soup, skim it.

16 **Avoid butter by cooking in your flavor.** You won't need to add butter to breads, pancakes, muffins, and other carb-based foods if you add herbs to breads, blueberries to pancakes, nuts and bananas to muffins. Grain-filled foods are often the ones that you most want to butter, but if you make them more flavorful, you can avoid the urge.

17 **Stock up on lemon pepper.** This seasoning adds wonderful flavor, not sodium, to your vegetables, meats, and starches. Use it freely as a salt substitute.

18 **Put an X on your calendar six weeks from now.** We are born with our preference for sugar, but salt is an acquired taste learned from habit. It takes about six weeks to "unlearn" your preference. Slowly reduce your intake of salt between now and then, focusing on food categories where the salt will be missed the least, such as cereals, breads, and dessert items. With this gradual decrease you won't get discouraged.

19 **Keep table salt in a small bowl with a tiny spoon.** To use far less of it, you can also use a pinch of your fingers to season your food. Cover it with a snug lid or some plastic wrap to keep it dry and less accessible.

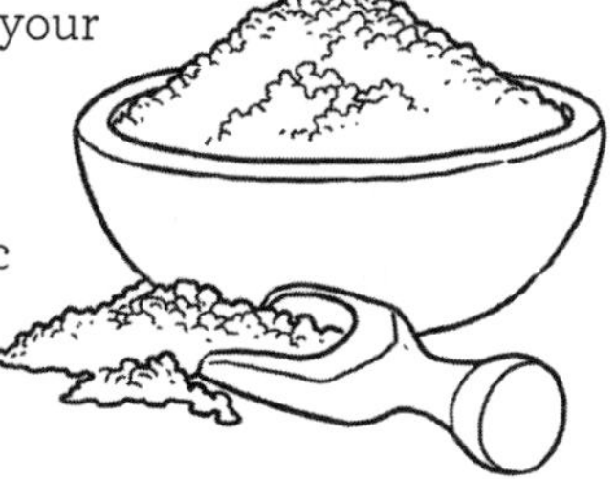

20 **Make your own salt-free salad dressing.** Mix one cup olive oil, one-third cup balsamic vinegar, one package sweetener, and two crushed garlic cloves in a bowl. Blend until emulsified. This keeps in the refrigerator for a month. Just remove an hour before serving so it can liquefy.

21 **Substitute citrus juice for salt in salad dressings.** Orange or lemon juice work well for this purpose.

22 **Have bacon!** A strip of bacon, cooked thoroughly, has fewer calories than a typical breakfast sausage link. Your best bet, though, is a slice of Canadian bacon—fewer calories and much less fat than the American type.

23 **Prep meals ahead of time.** Try easy-to-double recipes like lasagna, meatballs (make 'em with turkey to reduce the heart-clogging saturated fat), lentil soup, roast chicken, and eggplant casserole. Fill your freezer with the extras, and you will have healthy food handy when you are crunched for time.

24 **Always start with mirepoix.** This blend of onions, celery, carrots, parsley, and bay leaves (pronounced "meer-pwah") is a great way to sneak veggies into nearly every entrée you prepare. Sauté a cup (or more) of the mixture in two tablespoons of olive oil, then use a starter for sauces, stews, and soups.

25 **Look for high ORAC scores.** ORAC stands for oxygen radical absorbance capacity—a fancy way of answering "Which fruits and vegetables pack the greatest antioxidant punch?" According to the Agricultural Research Service's Human Nutrition Research Center on Aging at Tufts University in Boston, the top ten are: prunes, raisins, blueberries, blackberries, strawberries, raspberries, plums, oranges, red grapes, and cherries.

26 **Put salsa on your baked potato, not butter or sour cream.** You not only skip the fat but add in a healthy, low-cal serving of vegetables.

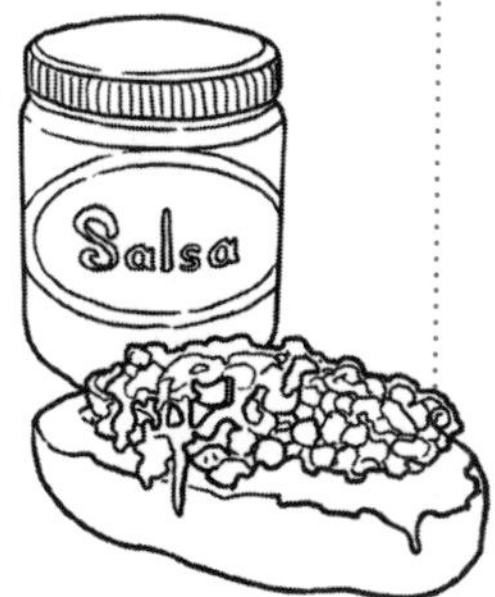

27 **Get some kind of vegetable and/or fruit with every fast-food meal.** Many fast-food restaurants now offer fruit instead of fries, or salads. You can also ask for extra tomatoes or lettuce on sandwiches.

28 **Choose biscotti.** These twice-baked Italian delicacies are perfect for dunking and often are fewer calories than doughnuts or sticky rolls.

29 **Replace mayonnaise in summer salads.** Instead, use nonfat yogurt, sour cream, or a mustard vinaigrette.

30 **Limit vacation splurges.** Let's be honest, when on vacation, many of us use that to splurge on all the unhealthy food we have been avoiding during our normal life. Limit yourself to one food splurge a day. If you do more, the uniqueness and specialness of the splurges fade away.

31 **Keep portions consistent.** A perfect breakfast has three components: one serving of a whole grain carbohydrate, one serving of a dairy or high-calcium food, and one serving of fruit; roughly 300 calories. A high-protein serving (a meat or an egg) is unnecessary but acceptable, as long as it doesn't add too much fat or calories. Two percent or whole milk may be more healthful than skim milk because it digests more slowly, giving a longer-lasting full feeling.

32 **Have a smoothie.** Whip up a cup of strawberries and a banana in the blender, add a scoop of protein powder and a cup of crushed ice, and you've got a healthy breakfast filled with antioxidants. Toss in a cup of plain yogurt, and you've just added a bone-strengthening dose of calcium. An added bonus: you've just crossed three of your daily fruit servings off the list.

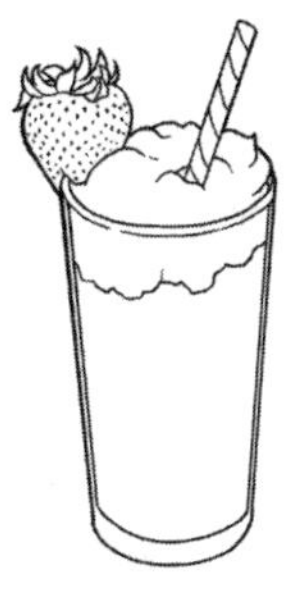

33 **Use butter substitutes.** They can significantly lower your total cholesterol level. These soft food spreads contain heart-healthy plant stanols (some examples are Benecol or Smart Balance). Just two tablespoons in place of butter can make a meaningful reduction in arterial plaque. Consider olive oil, coconut, or avocado oil spreads. Check the label: avoid products with a long list of ingredients, and make sure to avoid partially hydrogenated oils.

34 **Make your own granola bars.** Mix two cups rolled oats with one cup dried fruits and seeds and a little brown sugar. Toast three to five minutes in a warm oven and store in an airtight container. If you're not interested in do-it-yourself, there are a few store-bought brands (Nature's Path and Familia) with reasonable sugar and fat levels.

35 **Make the switch to high-fiber cereals.** These will provide the 25–30 grams of fiber you should be eating every day. People who start their day with a bowl of cold cereal get more fiber and calcium, but less fat, than those who breakfast on other foods. Those who ate two bowlfuls of high-fiber cereal every day cut the amount of fat consumed by 10 percent.

36 **Build your own sundae, any day.** Create a selection of sliced fruit, plain yogurt, whole grain cereals, and/or whole grain pancakes or toast, and let everyone mix and match to create their own toppings. Who says breakfast has to be boring?

37 **Eat an apple a day.** Apple slices with peanut butter provide a good start to the day. The protein and fat in the peanut butter are healthful, while the apple and the quercetin it contains provide fiber and protection against some cancers and heart disease.

38 **Find healthy proteins in the vegetarian section.** Soy bacon and sausage, Impossible Burgers, and mycoprotein (available in the brand Quorn), and other plant-based substitutes make great sources of protein for breakfast without the saturated fat of their meat originals. And remember, broccoli has more protein per calorie than steak.

39 **Make a grab-and-go breakfast.** Mix a half cup peanut butter, a quarter cup nonfat dry milk, three cups crushed flake cereal, and two tablespoons honey. Form into "blobs" (should make ten). Wrap each blob in plastic wrap and refrigerate. Grab a couple with a travel cup of milk and go!

40 **Increase your orange juice consumption.** The vitamin C in OJ boosts your immunity and improves your cholesterol levels. Three glasses of orange juice a day for four weeks can raise levels of HDL, or "good" cholesterol, by 21 percent. If three cups are too much, substitute a couple of oranges. For the healthiest effect, make it calcium-fortified juice.

41 **Serve up some pickled herring for breakfast or lunch.** This fish is rich in omega-3 fatty acids, shown to reduce inflammation and alleviate pain from arthritis and other joint diseases.

42 **Plant at least one vegetable.** You'll be more likely to eat it. Also plant some herbs to use in place of salt for flavoring food.

43 **Take advantage of prepared veggies.** Prepared foods are usually more expensive and high in artificial flavorings, sugars, and sodium. But we're all for prepared veggies—bagged salads, prewashed spinach, peeled and diced butternut squash, or washed and chopped kale. We're more likely to use bagged salads and other produce.

Order your pizza with extra veggies. Instead of the same old pepperoni and onions, do your health and digestion a favor and try artichoke hearts, broccoli, hot peppers, and other exotic vegetables many pizza joints stock these days for their gourmet pies.

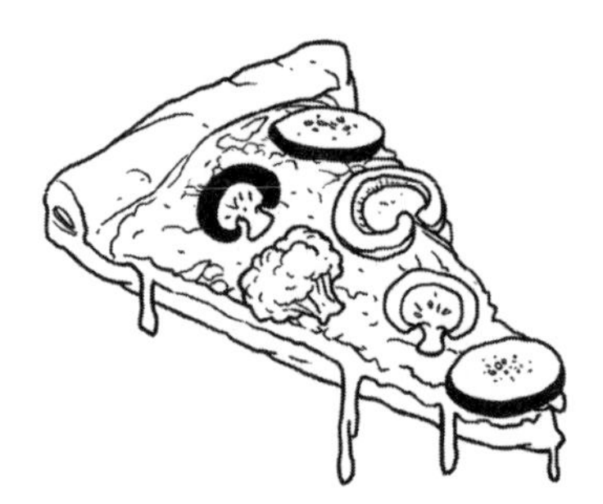

45 **Make a dinner rule: half of your plate should be vegetables.** That leaves a quarter of the plate for a healthful carb and a quarter for lean meat or fish. This makes the perfectly balanced dinner.

46 **Go exotic.** Try one new vegetable, fruit, meat, and/or grain every week. You may find a new favorite!

47 **Designate each weekday for a different-colored fruit.** Monday—Red: apples, cherries. Tuesday—Orange: apricots, cantaloupes. Wednesday—Yellow or White: bananas, yellow apples, grapefruit. Thursday—Blue or Violet: blueberries, blackberries, black raspberries. Friday—Green: limes, pears, kiwi.

48 **Switch one white food to a brown food each week.** Instead of instant white rice, switch to instant brown rice. Instead of regular pasta, switch to whole wheat pasta. Similarly, whole wheat pitas instead of regular, whole wheat tortillas instead of corn, whole wheat couscous instead of regular. Within two months, you should be eating only whole grains and should have increased your daily fiber consumption by an easy 10 grams without radically changing your diet!

49 **Wrap your food in lettuce leaves.** Skip the bun, tortillas, and bread slices and instead make a sandwich inside lettuce leaves. Go Mexican with a sprinkle of cheddar cheese, salsa, and chicken; Asian with sesame seeds, peanuts, bean sprouts, cut-up green beans, and shrimp with a touch of soy sauce; or deli style with turkey, cheese, and mustard.

50 **Buy old-fashioned snacks in kid-size bags.** Pretzels, tortilla chips, potato chips, and cookies are mostly bad carbs, made primarily of refined flour, sugar, salt, and/or oil. If you can't live without them, buy them in 1-ounce "lunch box" size and limit yourself to just one bag a day.

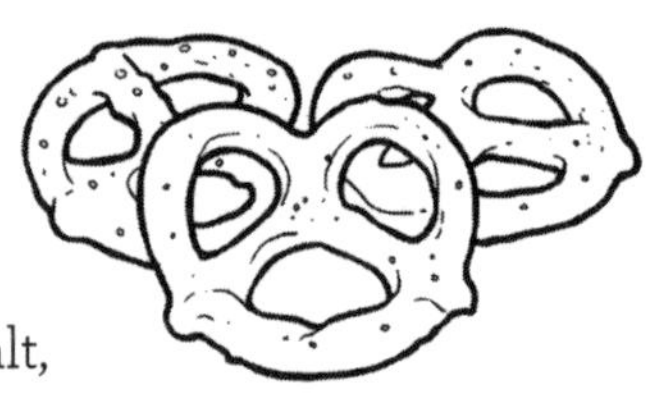

51 **Mix 1-ounce portions of cheese with 1-ounce portions of nuts.** Place into tiny snack bags for a handy snack at the ready.

52 **Establish rules about dessert.** For instance, have dessert only after dinner, never lunch. Eat dessert only on odd days of the month, or only on weekends, or only at restaurants. If you have a long tradition of daily desserts, then make it your rule to have raw fruit at least half the time.

53 **Make your own "sun tea" instead of lemonade.** Steep decaffeinated tea bags in water and set the pitcher in the sun for a couple of hours. Add lemon, lots of ice, and a sugar substitute for a carb-free summer quaff.

54 **Buy sugar-free condiments at the grocery store.** One tablespoon of ketchup can contain about half a teaspoon sugar, so buying sugar-free condiments can make a big dent in your carb consumption. Most condiments and other packaged foods for diabetics are made without sugar or with sugar substitutes.

55 **Remember these code words found on ingredient lists.** The only way to know if the processed food you're buying contains sugar is to know its many aliases or other forms. Here are the common ones: brown sugar, corn syrup, dextrin, dextrose, fructose, fruit juice concentrate, galactose, glucose, high-fructose corn syrup, honey, hydrogenated starch, invert sugar maltose, lactose, mannitol, maple syrup, molasses, polyols, raw sugar, sorbitol, sorghum, sucrose, turbinado sugar, and xylitol.

56 **If you must eat sweets, eat them with meals.** The other foods will help increase salivary flow, thus clearing the sugary foods from your mouth faster and helping prevent cavities. Of course, this does nothing for the calories you're imbibing and won't affect your weight, but at least you'll have a healthier mouth.

57 **Try all-fruit spread.** Sweet as sugar, but without the added sugar of jam, all-fruit spreads are wonderful not just on toast but melted into hot tea, mixed into cottage cheese or plain yogurt, and drizzled onto pancakes and waffles instead of syrup. Heat for ten seconds in the microwave to make it syrupy.

58 **Doctor your recipes with applesauce or pureed prunes.** Substitute for half the sugar in recipes. You can also use them in place of the recipe's fat.

59 **Choose sat-fat-free spreads.** You can find butter-like spreads in your refrigerated sections

that are low or even free of all saturated and trans fats, and actually taste good. Good brands to try include: Benecol (which will also help lower your cholesterol when used regularly), Canoleo, Earth Balance Pressed Avocado Oil, and Blue Bonnet. All except Blue Bonnet are trans-fat free; Blue Bonnet has 0.5 mg trans-fat per serving.

60 **Buy a pretty bottle, fill it with olive oil, and then top it with a liquor stop.** You know, the kind you use to pour out shots of liquor. Keep the bottle handy and use it for everything short of frying, because it burns at high temperatures. Olive oil is the best because it contains high amounts of monounsaturated fats and low amounts of saturated fats (all oils contain a mixture of the three: mono, poly, and saturated; the key is the ratio), isn't too strongly flavored, and is affordable. Buy the deepest green, extra virgin olive oil you can find—the darker the color, the greater the amount of phytonutrients, potent little plant-based cancer fighters.

61 **If you must have butter, mix it with olive oil.** Let a stick of butter soften at room temperature, beat the butter smooth, then slowly mix in a quarter- or half-cup of olive oil. You've just significantly cut the amount of saturated fat while adding loads of healthy monounsaturated fat.

62 **Eat the right meats.** Meat is one of the primary forms of saturated fat, but whether red or white, is also an excellent source of protein and trace minerals like zinc and iron. The key is choosing the right one. Of the nineteen cuts of beef that meet the USDA's labeling guidelines for lean, twelve have only 1 more gram of saturated fat on average than a comparable 3-ounce cooked serving of skinless chicken. The best choices include top sirloin beef, with 2.4 grams of saturated fat, and chuck pot roast, with 3 grams of saturated fat.

63 **Don't use cream to thicken soups.** Puree a cooked potato and an onion for the same, but healthier, effect.

64 **Use avocados in place of butter and cream.** These green fruits are called butter fruit in Mexico because they mash up into the same creamy texture as butter. Try them in soups as a thickening agent, and in mashed potatoes to provide a creamier texture as well as an added taste treat. Avocados and olives are the only two fruits high in fat, yet both are rich in heart-healthy monounsaturated fat.

65 **Substitute soy for meat or cheese at least once a week.** Soy cheese, soy burgers, and soy crumbles (like ground meat) are a great way to cut the saturated fat while retaining some semblance of the original food. Soy products may not be gourmet, but you can certainly handle the switch once a week.

66 **Give your canned veggies and beans a shower.** By rinsing under running water before cooking, you will get rid of much of the extra sodium.

67 **Watch out for salty condiments.** Capers, pickles, and olives are packed with salt. The pickling and brining processes used to make these foods primarily involves soaking them in a solution dense with salt.

68 **Avoid dried or cured meats.** These include beef jerky, salami, corned beef, prosciutto, ham, and dried sausages. They are dense with the salt used to draw out the liquid and preserve the meat. If you like meat snacks, turkey jerky has far less salt than beef.

FRUITS AND VEGGIES

1 **Start dinner with a mixed green salad.** Having this before the main course not only will help you eat more veggies. But by filling your stomach first with a nutrient-rich, low-calorie salad, there'll be less room for the higher-calorie items that follow.

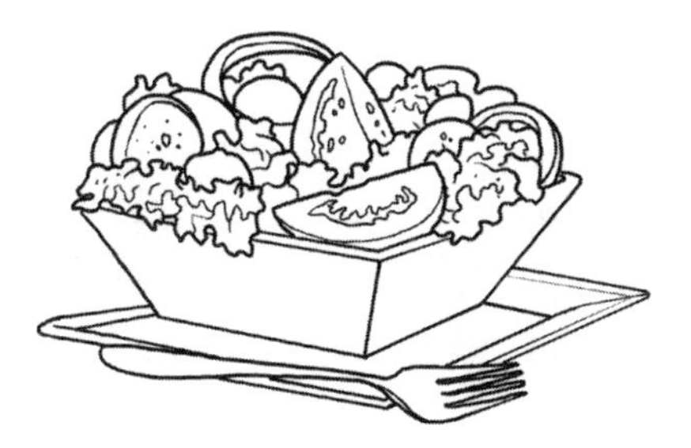

2 **Once a week, have a "whole meal" salad.** A Niçoise salad is a good example: mixed greens, steamed green beans, boiled potatoes, sliced hard-boiled egg, and tuna drizzled with vinaigrette. Serve with crusty whole grain bread.

3 **Energize your spaghetti sauce with vegetables.** Try a jar of low-sodium prepared sauce and add in green beans, peas, carrots, bell peppers, mushrooms, tomatoes, and more. If you like it chunky, cut them in big pieces, but if you don't want to know they're there, shred or puree them with a bit of sauce in the blender.

4 **Puree veggies into soup.** Just about any cooked vegetable can be made into a creamy, comforting soup. Here's one simple recipe: In a medium saucepan, sauté one cup finely chopped onion in one tablespoon olive oil until tender. Combine the onion in a blender or food processor with cooked vegetables and puree until smooth. Return puree to saucepan and thin with broth or low-fat milk, simmer, and season to taste.

5 **Add a bit of sweetness to your veggies.** A study found that students like broccoli and cauliflower more when the vegetables had a 5 percent sugar solution added to them (basically, just a bit of sugar or honey dissolved in water).

6 **Have a veggie burger for lunch at least once a week.** When topped with a sliced tomato and lettuce they taste better than you imagine.

7 **Open a can of low-sodium soup.** Add a bag of precut broccoli and carrots, either fresh or frozen. This makes a superfast and easy lunch or dinner entrée, ready to be flavored with your preferred spices, herbs, or hot sauce. As the soup simmers, it will simultaneously cook the veggies, boosting the nutritional value and fiber.

8 **Make your veggies top-shelf items.** As long as they are bagged properly, they'll last as well on the top shelf of the refrigerator as in a vegetable crisper. More important, now they'll be visible and enticing. Keep fast-to-eat vegetables like baby carrots, precut red and green pepper strips, broccoli or cauliflower florets, tomatoes, and cucumbers as accessible as possible.

9 **Eat vegetables like fruit.** A cucumber half, whole tomato, stalk of celery, or carrot are as pleasant to munch on as an apple. It may not seem typical, but who cares? A whole vegetable makes a terrific snack.

10 **Have a vegetable juice.** Although higher in sodium, vegetable juices, such as V8, do provide the nutrition of a vegetable serving. Throw a 6-ounce can of vegetable juice or tomato juice into your tote in the morning; many come in low-sodium forms.

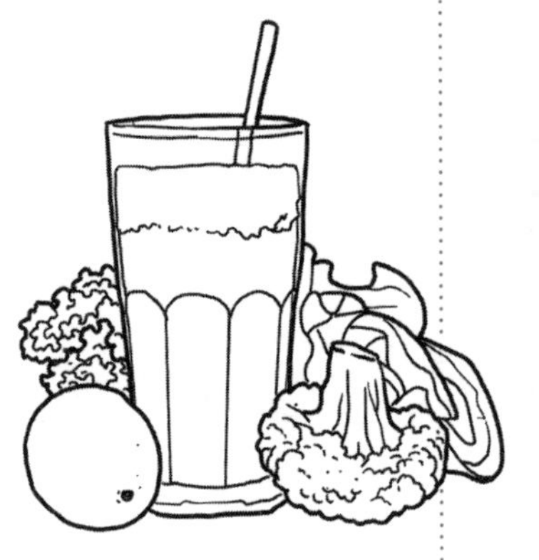

11 **Scoop out a tomato or green pepper.** Serve chili, soup, stew, pastas, or rice in them. Then you can eat the "bowl."

12 **Soup up your soup.** By adding chopped kale or other hearty greens to your next soup or stew, you will add potassium, fiber, and calcium. Just a couple of minutes is all that's needed to steam the greens down to tenderness.

13 **Vegetable juice up your soup.** Use low-sodium vegetable juice as the base for soups instead of chicken or beef broth.

14 **Be a vegetarian one day each week.** You can do this by merely substituting the meat serving with a vegetable serving like a crunchy, strong-flavored vegetable such as broccoli. You can dabble in the world of vegetarian cooking, in which recipes are developed specifically to make a filling, robust meal out of vegetables and whole grains. For those times, you should get yourself a quality vegetarian cookbook, such as *The Moosewood Cookbook,* which is popular for good reason. Other options are available online.

15 **Use salsa liberally.** Make sure you have a large batch filled with vegetables. You can add chopped yellow squash and zucchini to store-bought salsa. Then put it on things like baked potatoes, rice, chicken breasts, sandwiches, eggs, steak, even bread. It's too tasty and healthful not to be used all the time, instead of just on chips.

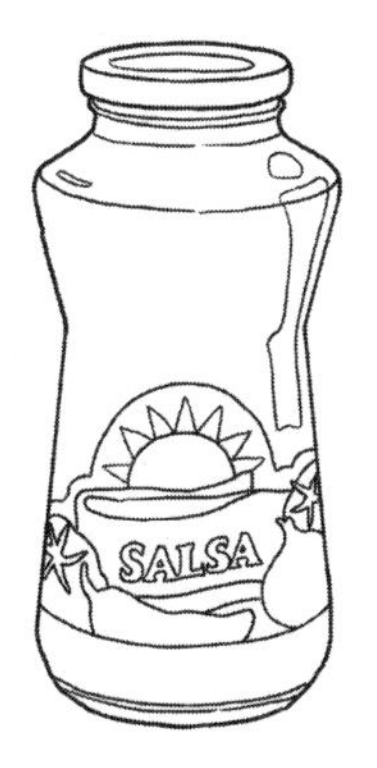

16 **Shredded carrots and cabbage are versatile.** They can be used in soups, salads, or casseroles. These coleslaw ingredients add flavor, color, and lots of vitamins and minerals.

17 **Use vegetables as sauces.** Try pureed roasted red peppers seasoned with herbs and a bit of lemon juice, then drizzled over fish. Or puree butternut or acorn squash with carrots, grated ginger, and a bit of brown sugar for a yummy topping for chicken or turkey. Cooked vegetables are easily converted into sauces with a little ingenuity and a blender.

18 **Salt away the bitterness of healthy veggies.** The chemical reality is that salt helps neutralize bitterness. For an added kick, try capers, olives, or mashed anchovies instead of salt.

19 **Grill your vegetables.** Peppers, zucchini, asparagus, onions, eggplant—even tomatoes—all taste great when grilled. All you need to do is coat them with olive oil, throw them on, turn every few minutes, and remove when they start to soften. Or skewer chunks of veggies on a bamboo or metal skewer and turn frequently. You can also buy grilling baskets that keep the veggies from falling through the slats in the grill.

20 **Make a new rule: Every breakfast should include a piece of fruit.** It's the perfect morning food, filled with natural, complex sugars for slow-release energy, fiber, and nutrients galore. Cantaloupe, an orange, berries—all are perfect with whole wheat toast, cereal, or an egg.

21 **Make another rule: Fruit for dessert at least three nights per week.** A slice of watermelon, a peach, or a bowl of blueberries can be the perfect ending to a meal, and are much more healthful than cookies or cake. If you like your desserts fancier, try chocolate-covered strawberries, poached pears in red wine, peach and blueberry crisp, or frozen fresh raspberry yogurt.

22 **Start your week with a fruit smoothie.** Add one cup of fresh fruit, a half cup of fruit juice, and one cup of ice to a blender and liquefy. That's two servings of fruit before 8:00 a.m.! If you'd prefer a creamier smoothie, toss in a half cup plain nonfat yogurt or kefir.

23 **Substitute fruit sorbet for ice cream.** One scoop (a quarter cup) contains up to one serving of fruit. To whip up your own, try freezing peaches packed in their own juice for twenty-four hours, then submerge the can in hot water for one minute. Cut the fruit into chunks and puree until smooth.

24 **Substitute frozen fruit bars for ice cream.** Buy pure-fruit versions that don't add extra corn syrup or sugar. Feel free to have one every single day.

25 **Keep a fruit bowl filled wherever you spend the most time.** This could be at work, near your home computer, or even in the television room. Keep five to eight pieces of fresh fruit in it at all times, such as bananas, oranges, apples, grapes, or plums. Most fruit is fine left at room temperature for three or four days, but if it's out and staring at you, it likely won't last that long. A piece of fruit makes a perfect snack—as often as four times per day.

26 **Get dried fruits to increase portability and shelf life.** Take them to work, on shopping trips, or on vacation. Raisins and prunes are classic choices. Try dried cranberries and blueberries, which are extremely high in phytonutrients, or dried apricots, which are rich in beta-carotene. Other options include dates, figs, dried peaches, dried pears, and dried bananas.

27 **If driving more than one hour, bring fruit with you.** Once you are on the highway and cruising along, an apple or nectarine tastes great and helps break the tedium.

28 **On long walks, keep an apple in your pocket.** It will be your reward for getting to the midpoint of your walk.

29 **Substitute prune puree or applesauce for oil in baking.** This works particularly well for brownies.

30 **Make a fruity salad.** A sprinkle of raisins, cut-up strawberries, diced apple, or sliced kiwi all make great additions to the typical tossed salad.

31 **Puree fresh or canned fruits.** Among others, you can use peaches, pears, mangoes, or apricots to use as an ice cream or pancake topping.

Use fresh or frozen berries in cereal, salads, or ice cream. They're also great stirred into yogurt or pancake and muffin mixes.

Freeze banana slices or grapes. This brings out their sweetness for a refreshing summer snack.

Substitute a small box of raisins for that candy bar. Raisins are sweet and healthful, and small boxes are just the right amount to fulfill a yen for a sweet treat.

Fruit-fortify your pancake or waffle batter. Fruits like strawberries, blueberries, and bananas will make your pancakes or waffles more enticing. The fruit can also be diced over these frozen breakfast items.

36 **Once a week, treat yourself to fruit in bread or cake.** How about pineapple upside-down cake,

applesauce cake, banana bread, strawberry, apple, or blueberry pie?

37 **Use orange juice as a base for cooking whole grains.** This will give your dish an unexpected and much-appreciated flavor boost.

38 **Spice up store-bought salsas with fruit.** Or make your own fruit-based salsas with pineapple, mango, or papayas. Mix with onions, ginger, a bit of garlic, some mint and/or cilantro, sprinkle on a few hot pepper flakes if desired, and chill.

39 **Make your salads special.** By adding diced kiwi, sliced grapes, or chopped apple to chicken, tuna, and turkey salads, you can impress your family or guests.

40 **For versatility, keep cut-up melon in the fridge.** Use as a first course before dinner, wrap with prosciutto for an appetizer, mix with cottage cheese for breakfast, or have a small bowl for a snack. Consider pureeing for a quick sauce over fish.

41 **Shred fresh fruit over plain yogurt.** Use the large holes of a cheese grater.

IN THE GARDEN

1 **Stretch for five minutes before heading out to the garden.** Focus on your hamstrings, back, and arms.

2 **Dress for gardening.** That means wearing sunscreen of SPF 30 or higher and reapplying it every couple of hours. Also put on bug repellant, a hat, sunglasses, and a light, long-sleeved shirt that covers most of your neck.

3 **Keep the local Poison Control hotline number handy.** Keep it by the telephone and with your gardening supplies in case you or someone near you is bitten by a snake or contaminated with pesticides or other garden chemicals.

4 **Bend with your knees.** Take frequent breaks from bending over. Back strain is a common gardening injury. Other good options to avoid strain are to carry a small stool with you to sit or lean on while weeding, and to use kneepads to protect your kneecaps from rocks and hard ground.

5 **Check the pollen index before heading outdoors.** This is particularly important if you suffer from allergies or asthma. Also, forgo gardening on days of high heat and humidity, when many areas issue ozone alerts. The heavy air could cause problems if you have any respiratory issues.

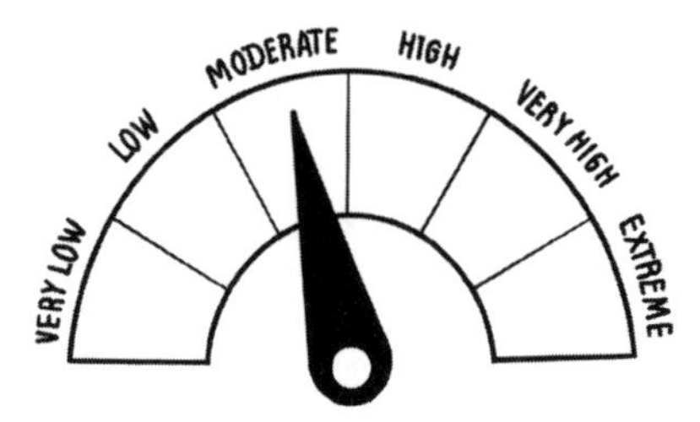

6 **Protect the joints in your hands and fingers.** Choose gardening tools with padded handles to avoid excess pressure. Tools like shears or clippers

with a spring-action, self-opening feature are particularly helpful if you have a weak grasp.

7 **Divide large, heavy bags into smaller loads.** Mulch, dirt, and fertilizer come in large, unwieldy bags that should be divided into smaller, more manageable loads. Use a cart or wagon to move heavy materials. When lifting, use the muscles in your legs, not your back.

8 **Avoid overstressing any one body part.** Vary your tasks. For instance, don't spend the entire day stooping and weeding. Instead, pick one section of the garden to weed, then lay mulch and rake. Tackle another section the following day.

9 **Use a backpack or tool belt.** Keep all your gardening tools, gloves, and so on in something you can carry with you as you move around the garden.

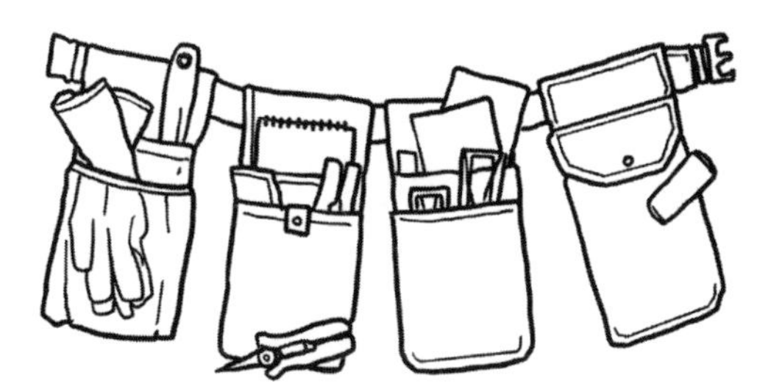

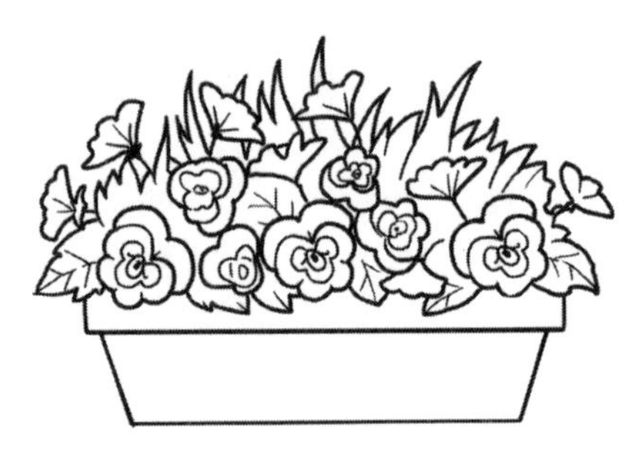

10 **Keep your garden manageable.** That might even mean container gardening. If you take on too much too soon, not only will you find yourself sore the next morning (and risk a more serious injury), but you'll quickly become overwhelmed and quit altogether.

11 **Keep a water bottle handy.** Be sure to sip on it every thirty minutes or so. It's easy to become dehydrated when you're working in the yard.

EXCELLENT EXERCISE

1. **Hydrate on your way to the gym.** Drink a bottle of water before you arrive. If you show up for your workout dehydrated, you'll feel overly fatigued during your session. By arriving at the gym hydrated you work harder, you feel more energized, and your mental function is alert, so you get much more out of your workout.

2. **Work out with a friend.** If you often think of skipping your workouts, ask a friend to meet you for a gym date. As you walk or run on the treadmill, you can share stories of your day and the time will fly by quickly. You can also encourage each other to work a bit harder. Your friend can also help you find the courage to approach unfamiliar gym equipment, as it's easier

to laugh off your foibles when you have a trusted companion nearby.

3 **Slow down.** People who lift weights slowly—taking at least fourteen seconds to complete one repetition—gained more strength than those who lifted at a rate of seven seconds per repetition. Slower lifting may help increase strength because it prevents you from using momentum or cheating with improper technique.

4 **Take a Pilates class once a week.** Developed by Joseph Pilates in the early 1920s, this regimen places a heavy emphasis on the abdominals and core as it simultaneously strengthens the arms and legs. Although many books and videos teach the Pilates method, you'll have best results by taking a few classes from a certified instructor. Once you learn the basic technique, you can then practice at home with a video.

5 **Stretch during TV time.** Sprawl out on the floor and go through your stretching routine. If you feel good, do them a second or even a third time. It's best to do this later in the day, when your muscles are warmed up from your daily activities.

6 **While driving, tighten your tummy and pelvic floor muscles.** Starting with your pubic area, begin to tighten from the bottom up. Once you squeeze your pelvic floor, suck your lower belly and then upper belly in toward your spine as you exhale. Hold for a count of five, then release and repeat ten to twenty times.

7 **Do donkey kicks when you feel tired.** Stand up, place your palms on your desk, bend one knee, flex that foot, and kick your leg back, as if you were a donkey kicking someone behind you. Alternate legs for fifteen total kicks. Then return to work refreshed and with a stronger backside.

8 **Take the stairs two or three at a time.** Similar to a traditional step-up exercise done at the gym, this strengthens the gluteal muscles in your buttocks and revs up your heart rate, boosting your cardiovascular fitness.

9 **Do the "lunge walk" to the mailbox.** During each step forward to the mailbox, bend your knees and sink down until both legs form ninety-degree angles. Then press into your front heel to rise. Lift your back leg and knee all the way into your chest

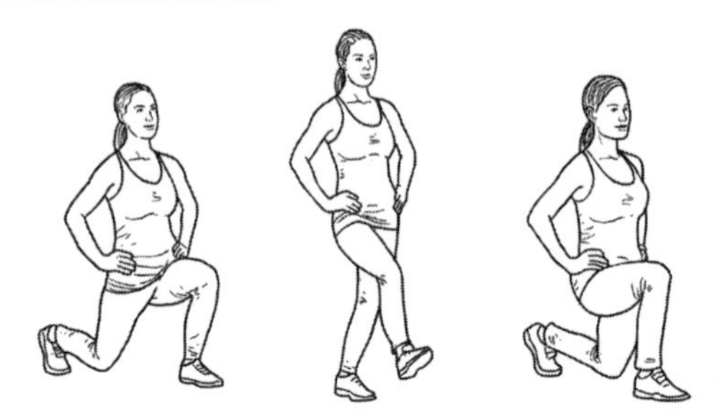

before planting it in front of you for the next lunge. This will take a little practice, but if you do this "lunge walk" for twenty or more steps a day, your legs will be far stronger and shapelier.

10 **Do chair crunches.** Sit on the edge of your chair, lift your feet off the floor, bringing your knees into your chest. Lower and repeat ten to fifteen times.

11 **When standing in line, lift one foot.** Stand on one leg and try to hold your balance. You'll feel myriad muscles in your abdomen and back firing up to help steady your body. Make sure to alternate your feet.

12 **Use your stability ball to do abs and back exercises.** At work or home, you can perform abdominal or back exercises on your new desk

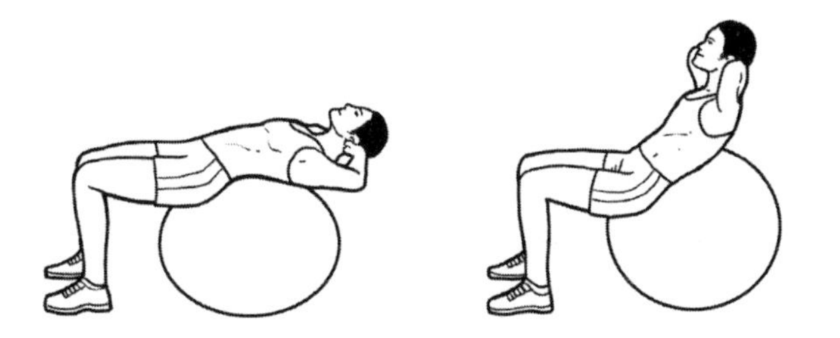

chair—uh, ball—that are nicely effective. When you perform abdominal-strengthening movements on a stability ball, you use more of your core muscles for every movement. Try the traditional crunch on the ball.

13 **For a simple, effective back stretch, lie flat on your back.** Lift one knee to your chest, then the other, keeping your lower back on the floor. Wrap your arms behind your knees, using them to support your legs and, if necessary, pulling them so your buttocks rise off the floor. You should feel your back muscles stretching. Hold the position for thirty seconds, then release.

14 **Try the reciprocal reach.** You can strengthen your abs and back at the same time with this exercise, also sometimes called "opposite limb extension." Three times per week, when you arrive home from work, get on all fours with your hands under your shoulders and knees under your hips. Extend your left leg behind, placing the ball of your left foot against the floor while tucking your tailbone and keeping it tucked throughout the exercise. Lift your left foot off the floor as you lift your right arm, reaching your right hand and left foot away from each other, keeping your hips level; hold for ten to twenty seconds, release, and repeat on the other side for two to three sets.

15 **Do leg lifts as you cook dinner.** Flex your foot and lift your leg out to the side, lower, and repeat ten to fifteen times. Then switch legs. You'll finish your leg workout before dinnertime.

16 **Whenever you feel exasperated at work, press your forehead into your palms.** Many people tense up their neck muscles when under stress, which can lead to pain and stiffness. Reduce tension and strengthen your neck at the same time with this simple exercise.

17 **Exercise your rotator cuff once a week.** Your rotator cuff is a group of muscles and tendons that hold your shoulder joint in place. Most people neglect to strengthen this area of the body because these deep muscles don't play much of a role in shaping sexy shoulder contours, and no one tells you about these muscles until after you've already injured them. At-home exercises and stretches will go a long way toward preventing shoulder problems later in life. Good news: most are quick and easy, such as the pendulum. Lean forward with one arm hanging freely. Use the other arm to brace yourself on a table or chair. Gently swing the hanging arm side to side, back and forth, and in a circular motion. Repeat on the other side.

18 Whenever you spend more than forty-five minutes in the driver's seat or in front of the computer, practice the "turtle" exercise.

During driving and staring at a computer screen, we tend to jut our heads forward, but the head weighs about ten pounds, so this puts quite a bit of stress on the back of the neck, leading to headaches. You can strengthen the muscles in the back of your neck and train yourself to sit with proper posture with the following exercise. As you drive or type, pretend you are a turtle retracting your head into your shell, keeping your chin level, bringing your head back, and flattening the curve in the back of your neck. Hold for a count of five, release, and repeat ten times.

19 **Roll your neck every hour.** Drop your chin to your chest, then roll your neck to the left, back, to the right, and down again in a circular motion. Repeat five times, then switch direction, starting with a roll to the right.

20 **Roll on a tennis ball whenever you feel tight.** If your foot feels tense, stand with one hand against a wall for support and place the arch of one foot on top of the ball. Gradually add more body weight over the foot, allowing the ball to press into your arch, then begin to slowly move your foot, allowing the ball to massage your heel, forefoot, and toes. If the tennis ball seems too big for your foot, try a golf ball instead. You can also lie on the ball to get at that hard-to-reach spot between the shoulder blades or to soothe tension in your low back, and for tight hips, sit on the ball, wiggling your booty around and holding it in any spot that feels particularly good.

21 **After wearing high heels all day, give your calves some attention.** Elevating your heels all day long can eventually shorten your calf muscles. To release them, sit on the floor with your knees bent and feet on the floor. Grasp one ankle, placing your thumb over your Achilles tendon, press your thumb into the bottom of your calf muscle, hold for five seconds, and release. Move an inch up your calf and repeat pressing and releasing until you get to your knee, then switch legs.

22 **Make your own hot massager with a tube sock.** Fill a tube-style athletic sock three-fourths full with uncooked rice, tie off the end tightly with a rubber band, and stick it in the microwave for two minutes. Remove the sock and rub it up and down your legs and arms for a gentle, soothing hot massage. Leave the sock filled with the rice; you can use it over and over. You can add spices to the rice if you wish to have a pleasant scent while massaging.

23 **Use interval training to rev up your workout.** Varying the intensity of your workout throughout your exercise session will burn more calories in the same amount of time, and prevent boredom that can set in by doing the same routine every day. Every five minutes into your walk, jog for one minute. Every five minutes into your bike ride, shift into a higher gear and pedal hard for a minute. If you swim, turn on the speed every other lap.

24 **Find a class or instructor you like.** Look for a teacher you can trust. Videos created by personal trainers and exercise physiologists (or classes taught by them) are more likely to motivate you than those hosted by supermodels or influencers.

25 **Release your neck whenever you're on hold.** Use the speakerphone or your headset, and the next time someone puts you on hold, do some neck rolls or get down on the floor and start doing your stretching routine.

26 **Shoot for 10,000 steps a day.** Don't let that amount scare you. Most people walk about 5,500 to 7,500 steps during an average day as they amble to and from meetings, to the watercooler, to the mailbox. In fact, researchers who study these types of things consider 5,000 steps a day a "sedentary lifestyle." According to researchers at Arizona State University in Mesa, you can cover 7,499 steps a day without participating in formal sports or exercise. If you garner 10,000 steps a day you're considered "active," while 12,500 steps a day garners you the title of "highly active." Using your pedometer/phone/Fitbit, find your baseline of how many steps you normally take a day. Then increase that amount by at least 200 steps a day until you reach 10,000 to 12,500 steps daily.

27 **Train for school fitness tests as a family.** Learn which fitness tests your child is required to pass in PE and train for them as a family. Set goals, such as running a quarter mile and then a half, and then a full mile in a certain amount of time. And reward all family members for meeting their goals.

28 **Do abdominal exercises as a warm-up for your workout.** The typical workout starts with five or ten minutes of walking or marching to get your body warmed up and the blood flowing. But let's face it, that's boring. Instead, do your abdominal work. Because your abdomen consists of large muscle groups, abdominal work is very warming for the body. Five to ten minutes of abdominal exercises will warm you up as well as a walk and give you some good muscle building at the same time.

29

Add some weight. Ankle weights, that is! One set of ankle weights allows you to do just about any leg exercise at home, and you'll never have to set foot in the gym again to maintain shapely legs. In addition to the traditional leg lifts, you can use ankle weights to do other leg exercises such as hamstring curls and leg extensions. Or just use them on your walks. Look for ankle weights that allow you to add weight as you get stronger, and with Velcro straps rather than shoelaces for easy access.

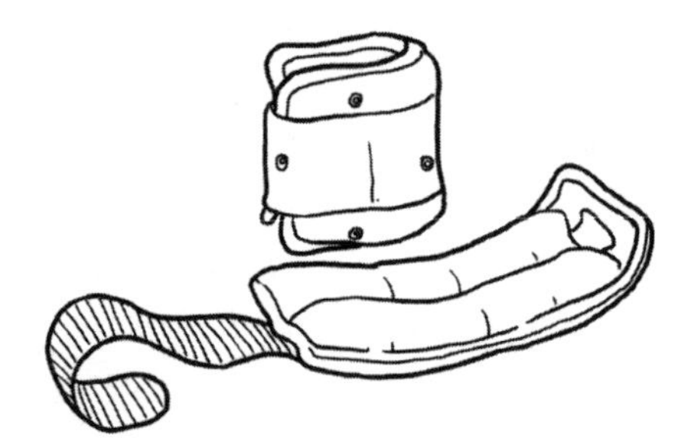

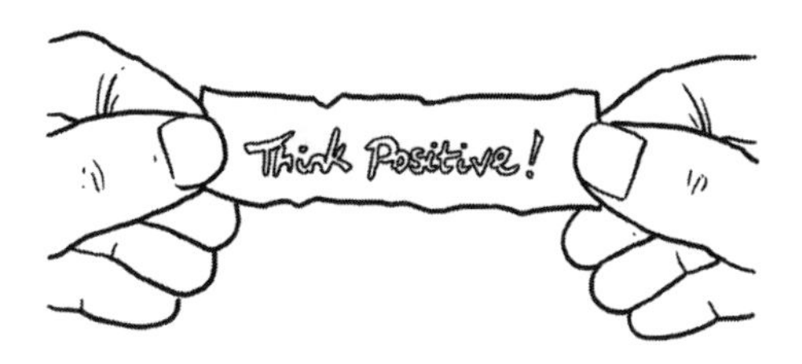

30 **Think you can and you will.** So often ignored, positive thinking can help you power your way through a workout. Exercisers who think positively are more likely to stay active than those whose minds often utter those two evil words: "I can't." Whenever you find yourself making excuses, put those self-defeating thoughts away in the back of your brain and replace them with positive messages such as, "I feel great," or "Bring it on."

31 **Be mindful as you move.** Rather than daydreaming through your workouts, put as much mental emphasis on what you do at the gym as you do at work. For example, when doing a strength exercise, feel the muscle contract as you lift. This inner focus will help you improve your technique. You'll fatigue your muscles faster because you'll make every movement count.

32 **Squeeze your butt when you walk.** Imagine you are holding a $50 bill between your butt cheeks, and as you firm and lift your buttocks muscles to hold your imaginary bill, you'll strengthen your back muscles. You can also work your abs as you walk by imagining you have a zipper along the midline of your abdomen. Picture yourself zipping up a tight pair of jeans, and as you pull the zipper up your abdomen, feel your torso lengthen and abdomen firm. Keep your abs zipped up and your butt clenched throughout your walks and you'll strengthen your core even as you burn fat.

33 **Add a hill to your walking route.** As you trudge up the hill, you'll feel the muscles in the backs of your legs working hard to push off with every step.

34 **Practice kickboxing moves for five minutes every morning before dressing.** There's nothing like seeing your bare thighs in the mirror to motivate you to do your kicks. Kick in all directions, mixing in front kicks, side kicks, back kicks, and roundhouse kicks. No matter what kick you do, never fully extend your knee. This protects your knee joint.

35 **Do the twist.** Whether you're on the dance floor at a wedding or in your living room tonight, bend your knees and squat down as far as you comfortably can as you shimmy from side to side. You'll burn calories, have a few laughs, and strengthen your legs at the same time.

36 **Jump into the pool once or twice a week.** Sports coaches have typically told their athletes to increase their leg strength through plyometrics, which are a series of skipping, jumping, and bounding exercises usually done on land. Because of the force of gravity and the impact of the body as it hits the ground, these exercises result in quite a bit of post-exercise muscle soreness, which is

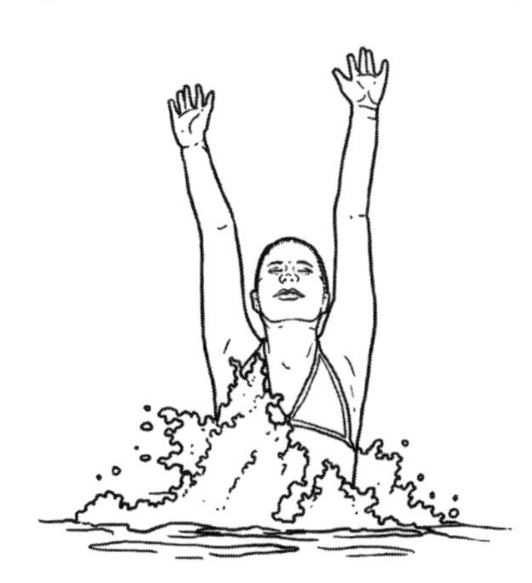

why we're not recommending you do them. If you complete the exercises in a swimming pool, you can get the leg-strength benefit from plyometrics without the post-exercise soreness.

37

Use a six- to eight-inch ball as an abdominal strengthening companion. Children's balls called Gertie balls or small, light fitness balls make great workout aids. Use one in the kitchen while cooking. Place the ball between your thighs, just above your knees. As you stir your food at the stove or chop vegetables, squeeze your inner thighs to hold the ball in place and fire up your pelvic floor and lower abdominal muscles.

38

Do shrugs with weights for upper-body strength. Hold a light dumbbell in each hand, allowing your arms to hang down naturally at your sides, palms facing in, with your legs about shoulder width apart. Slowly shrug your shoulders straight up toward your ears, pause, and then lower them back to starting position. Repeat until your muscles feel fatigued. Don't rotate your shoulders—that will strain them—instead, concentrate on going straight up and down.

39 **Do the torso twist.** This is easy, yet effective at building the oblique muscles that line the sides of your abdomen and improving your golf swing. Standing upright with your feet shoulder width apart, hold a broomstick or cardboard tube across your shoulders and behind your neck so it is resting on the top of your back, with your hands near the ends of the broomstick or tube. Keeping your hips as still as possible, smoothly twist to your left as far as you can go, moving your head with your torso (otherwise, you might strain your neck). Come back to the starting position, pause, then twist in the opposite direction, repeating at a slow, steady pace until you tire.

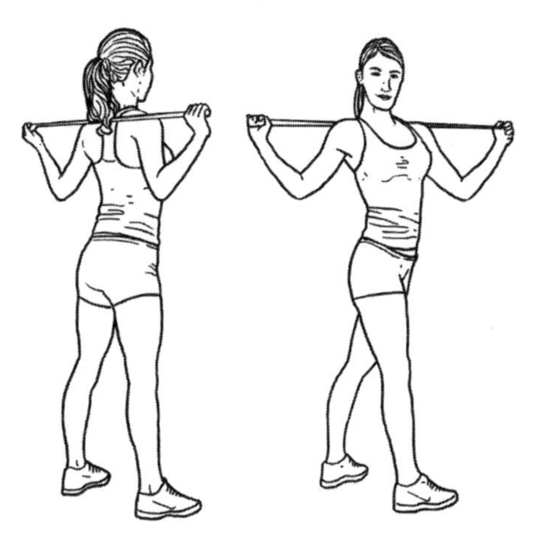

40 **Dance your way to flexibility.** Take a dance class once a week. Twenty cross-country skiers were tested for flexibility. Half of them took a dance class, while the other half served as a control group. Within three months, the skiers who took the weekly dance class improved the flexibility of their spines and increased their agility and ski speed on a slalom and hurdle test.

41 **Stretch during your shower routine.** The perfect time of day to sneak in a little stretching is right after—or during—a warm shower in the morning. Your muscles are warm and it is a great way to energize your day. Try the following routine: In the shower, raise your arms above your head, clasp your hands, and reach upward to stretch your shoulders and back. With the water spray hitting the back of your neck, slowly turn your head to the right until your chin is over your shoulder. Pause, then slowly turn your head all the way to the left. Repeat five times in each direction. Dry off with one foot on the toilet, lean forward, and stretch your hamstring. While drying your hair, hold a calf stretch by extending one leg two to three feet behind the other.

42 **Take calisthenics breaks.** Whether working at the office or your home office, take a five- or ten-minute break every hour and do jumping jacks, lunges, push-ups, or crunches. Over the course of the day, you'll have exercised for more than sixty minutes—and finished that big project on time.

CALORIE CONTROL

1 **Fidget.** People who drum their fingers or bounce their knees burn at least an extra 500 calories a day! That adds up to losing a pound a week.

2 **Don't starve yourself.** Cutting too many calories can backfire in more ways than one. Try to subsist on morsels, and your metabolism will slow so much that you'll not only stop losing weight, but you'll be lucky if you can peel yourself off the couch.

3 **Keep a small squeeze ball handy.** Work out your hands frequently during the day. It's one of the few exercises you can do anytime. You'll build up the muscles in your hands and forearms—and muscle, whether in your hands or legs, burns a lot of calories.

4 **Once a week, indulge in a high-calorie-tasting, but low-calorie treat.** This should help keep you from feeling deprived and bingeing on higher-calorie foods. For instance: lobster—83 calories in 3 ounces; edamame—105 calories in a half-cup serving; apple slices with peanut butter—267 calories for a small apple with two tablespoons of peanut butter; whipped cream—8 calories in 1 tablespoon.

5 **Treat high-calorie foods as jewels in the crown.** Make a spoonful of ice cream the jewel and a bowl of fruit the crown. Cut down on the chips by pairing each bite with lots of chunky, filling fresh salsa. Balance a little cheese with a lot of salad.

6 **After breakfast, make water your primary drink.** At breakfast, go ahead and drink orange juice, but throughout the rest of the day, focus on water instead. The average American consumes an extra 245 calories a day from soft drinks, nearly 90,000 calories a year—or 25 pounds! Despite the calories, sugary drinks don't trigger a sense of fullness the way food does.

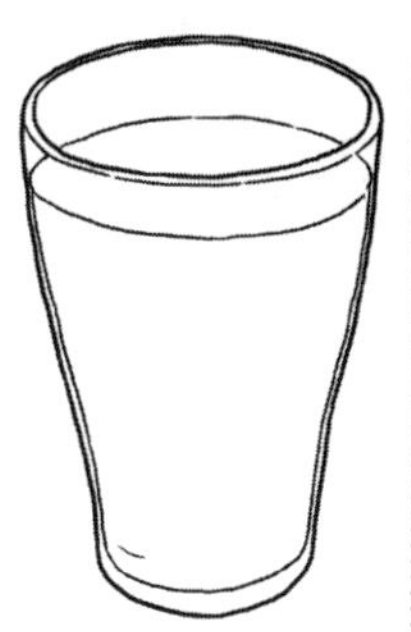

7 **Find an online weight-loss buddy.** They help you keep the weight off. An eighteen-month study showed those on an Internet-based weight maintenance program sustained their weight loss better than those who met face-to-face in a support group.

8 **Bring the color blue into your life more often.** The color blue functions as an appetite suppressant. So serve up dinner on blue plates, dress in blue while you eat, and cover your table with a blue tablecloth. Conversely, avoid red, yellow, and orange in your dining areas. Studies find they encourage eating.

9 **Downsize your dinner plates.** The less food put in front of you, the less you'll eat, and the converse is true—regardless of how hungry you are. Instead of using regular dinner plates that range these days from ten to fourteen inches, which look forlornly empty if they're not heaped with food, serve your main course on salad plates about seven to nine inches wide. The same goes for liquids. Instead of 16-ounce glasses and oversized coffee mugs, return to the old days of 8-ounce glasses and 6-ounce coffee cups.

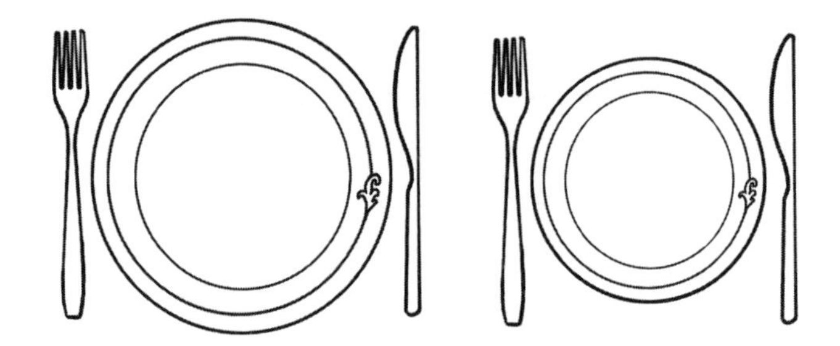

10 **Eat 90 percent of your meals at home.** You're more likely to eat more—and more high-fat, high-calorie foods—when you eat out than when you eat at home. Restaurants today serve such large portions that many have switched to larger plates and tables to accommodate them!

11 **Watch the first four ingredients on the label.** Avoid any prepared food that lists sugar, fructose, or corn syrup among the first four ingredients. You should be able to find a lower-sugar version of the same type of food. If you can't, grab a piece of fruit instead! Look for sugar-free varieties of foods such as ketchup, mayonnaise, and salad dressing.

12 **Eat slowly and calmly.** Put your fork or spoon down between every bite. Sip water frequently. Intersperse eating with stories of the amusing things that happened during your day. Your brain lags your stomach by about twenty minutes when it comes to satiety (fullness) signals, so if you eat slowly enough, your brain will catch up to tell you that you are no longer in need of food.

13 **Eat only when you hear your stomach growling.** It's stunning how often we eat out of boredom, nervousness, habit, or frustration—so often, in fact, that many of us have actually forgotten what physical hunger feels like. Next time wait until your stomach is growling before you reach for food. If you're hankering for a specific food, it's probably a craving, not hunger.

If you'd eat anything you could get your hands on, chances are you're truly hungry.

14 **Find ways other than eating to express love, tame stress, and relieve boredom.** You might make your family a photo album of special events instead of a rich dessert, sign up for a stress-management course at the local hospital, or take up an active hobby, like bowling.

15 **Minisize your sandwich.** When purchasing sandwiches from a deli or cafeteria, ask for a half portion. In one study, participants presented with a twelve-inch sandwich ate the entire thing but felt just as satisfied afterward as when they ate an eight-inch sandwich. Apparently seeing less translates into eating less.

16 **Have your cocktail after dinner, not before.** In a study conducted at the University of Liverpool in England, men who drank a glass of beer thirty minutes before a meal ate more during the meal than men who consumed a nonalcoholic beverage. They also ate more fatty, salty foods and felt hungrier after the meal than men who did not drink.

17 **Check the menu before you leave home.** Most restaurants have their menus on their websites, and many include calorie counts. You can decide before you ever hit the hostess stand what you're going to order. Conversely, if you don't see anything that's healthy, pick another restaurant.

18 **Turn up the heat with hot peppers.** Some studies show that very spicy foods can temporarily increase your metabolism. Gourmet groceries often stock a dozen different kinds of peppers. Buy one a week and practice adding some to various meals. Spice up your scrambled eggs with minced jalapeno, add a little fire to your beef stew with half a diced banana pepper, or pull together a spicy jambalaya (using turkey sausage and lots of veggies).

19 **Add 10 percent to the number of daily calories you think you are eating, then adjust your eating habits.** If you think you are consuming 1,700 calories a day and don't understand why you are not losing weight, add another 170 calories to your guesstimate. Chances are, the new number is more accurate.

WONDERFUL WALKS

1 **Learn the basics.** Before you take your next step outdoors, you need to know how much walking to do, and how often. Walk at a pace that has you breathing heavily, but still able to carry on a conversation. Your goal is to walk thirty minutes five days a week. Walking hard for thirty minutes can be difficult depending on your fitness level. Walk as long as you are comfortable the first week. Start every walk slowly for five minutes, then cool down at the end with another five minutes of easy-paced walking. When you reach the target of thirty minutes a day, five days a week, set a new target. Either increase your time, or try new forms of exercise, such as strength-building exercises twice a week.

2 **Walk with a friend.** If they're expecting you, you're more likely to get out of bed on cold winter mornings or skip the cafeteria for a lunchtime walk. If one of you backs out for any reason, put $5 in a kitty. Hopefully this will never happen, but if you manage to build up any substantial sum, donate it to charity.

3 **Walk for entertainment one day a week.** Instead of walking around your neighborhood, walk through the zoo, an art museum, or an upscale shopping mall. First circle the perimeter of your location at your usual brisk pace, then wander through more slowly to take in the sights.

4 **Use a Fitbit or other activity tracker.** They measure how far you've walked in steps and miles, and provide motivation by spurring you to meet a particular goal and whether you've met it. People who wore a Fitbit or other device automatically increased the number of steps they took in a day. Often, activity trackers hook onto your belt and are small and easy to use. Smartphone apps automatically record while going through repetitive motion in your pocket or strapped to your arm.

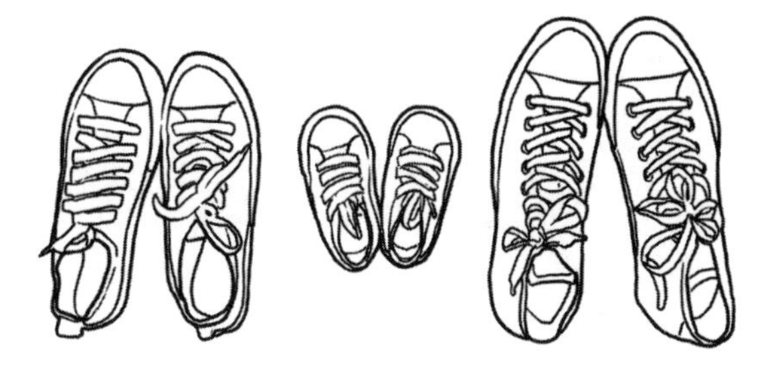

5 **Take the entire family on your daily walks.** Not only will you be modeling good fitness habits for your children, but you'll also be able to supervise them while you walk, rather than getting a sitter. If your children walk too slowly, ask them to ride their bikes or roller-skate alongside you. To keep everyone entertained, play your usual repertoire of long car trip games such as "I Spy." You can also try a scavenger walk, where you start out with a list of items to find during your walk and check off the list as you spot them.

6 **Once a week, complete your errands on foot.** If you live within a mile of town, or even a convenience store, start from your house. If you live out in the middle of nowhere, drive to within a mile of your destination, park, and walk the rest of the way there and back. You'll be surprised how much you can accomplish on foot and how many people you'll meet along the way.

7 **Improve your walking posture.** Proper posture will reduce discomfort and help you burn more fat and calories. Stand tall with your spine elongated and breastbone lifted. Keep your head straight with your eyes focused forward and shoulders relaxed. Roll your feet from heel to toe. As you speed up, take smaller, more frequent steps. Allow your arms to swing freely. Firm your tummy and flatten your back as you walk to prevent low back pain.

8 **Breathe deeply as you walk to a count of 1-2-3.** Many people unintentionally hold their breath when they exercise and then suddenly feel breathless and tired. Muscles need oxygen to create the energy for movement. As you inhale, bring the air to the deepest part of your lungs by expanding your ribs outward and your tummy forward and inhale for a count of three. Then exhale fully either through your nose or mouth, also to the count of three.

9 **Periodically pick up the pace.** Prevent boredom by keeping your mind and body engaged by periodically picking up the pace or challenging yourself by trudging up a hill. Every ten to fifteen minutes, complete a two- to three-minute surge. During your surge, try to catch a real or imaginary walker ahead of you.

10 **Pump up the volume.** People with severe respiratory disease who listened to music while walking covered four more miles during an eight-week study than a similar group who did not listen to music. Researchers speculate that listening to music made the participants feel less hindered by shortness of breath and distracted them from possible boredom and fatigue. You don't have to have lung disease to benefit from music during your walks, so bring along a headset and play your favorite tunes.

11 **When you don't feel like walking, promise yourself just ten minutes.** Once you've warmed up, you'll exercise for longer than you anticipated.

Even if you don't walk longer, ten minutes is better than no minutes at all.

12 **Walk in the evening.** After-dinner walks get you away from the television, keep you from eating too much at dinner, it's when your neighbors are outside, and it's just a lovely time of day. Don't let unlovely weather stop you either—that's what jackets, boots, and umbrellas were invented for. There's something childlike and fun about a walk in the rain or snow.

13 **If you're over sixty, walk on soft surfaces.** As you age, the fat padding in your feet deteriorates. The absence of this natural shock absorber can make walking on sidewalks and other hard surfaces feel like foot torture. Flat grass and dirt paths will provide more cushioning for your feet than roads or sidewalks.

14 **Train for an event.** Search online for fun runs and walks being held in your area. These events raise money for good causes and are great motivators. The Leukemia and Lymphoma Society offers a Team in Training program that will get you in marathon walking shape. The

society assigns you a coach and walking plan, and you raise money through donations. (If you can't attend an event in person for any reason, consider joining a virtual run or walk: register online, choose a starting point, cover the distance, and upload your time.)

15 **Apply some lube.** If you're a long-distance walker or somewhat overweight, chafing clothes can make you want to call it quits. You can solve the problem by wearing skin-hugging clothing and lubing up your sensitive areas with Vaseline or Waxelene, which acts like a barrier to protect your skin.

16 **Split it up.** When you're too busy to go for your usual thirty- or sixty-minute walk, split it up and get out there for five or ten minutes at a time. Taking a five-minute walk break around the building after completing a big project at work will refresh your mind, so you can return to work with more vigor. Most of us can focus at top capacity for only thirty minutes at a time. After that, concentration begins to drop off so your intermittent walk breaks may actually make you more productive.

17 **Walk as you talk.** Walk around the house with your cell phone as you chat with friends or conduct business. This is a great way to make use of those long hold times with the IRS, cell phone provider, or Internet service provider. Not only will you get some heart-healthy exercise, but it will help you maintain your mental cool. Your Fitbit or cell phone app can count your steps so you'll get the added bonus of feeling like you accomplished something rather than just wasting time.

18 **Walk faster earlier in your walk.** Some bursts of faster walking toward the beginning of your walk will increase the amount of fat burned. Many walkers wait until the end of the walk to speed up, treating it as a finishing kick. Exercisers burned more fat and felt less fatigued when they inserted their faster segments toward the beginning of a workout. It works because you speed up your heart rate early and keep it elevated for the rest of your walk.

19 **Give your walk some weight.** Carrying 3- to 5-pound weights builds muscle. Each pound of muscle burns about 30 to 50 more calories a day, so building a couple of pounds of muscle in your arms alone will burn an extra 100 calories a day even while you're just channel surfing. Isometric exercises of the arms, chest, and abdominal muscles can be done while you walk by simulating throwing a punch in slow motion while holding weights. As you extend your arm, tense the muscles along it and do the same as you retract it; you should feel tension in your triceps, biceps, deltoids, and pectoral muscles. Repeat with your arms going up and down, or out to the side, rather than straight ahead. Tense your chest muscles by bringing your hands together in front of your body and contracting across the chest and shoulders rhythmically to match your gait, or try doing curls with no weights by simply curling your arms alternately, in rhythm with your gait, and each time, tense your biceps.

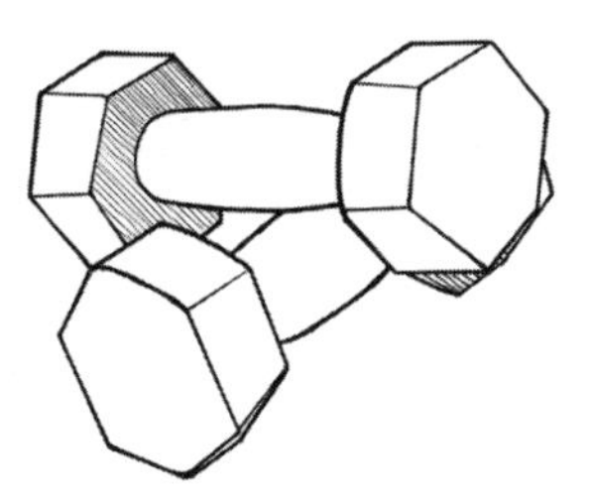

MAKING THE MOST OF WEEKENDS

1 **Get out of bed at the same time as during the week.** When you sleep in until noon, it's hard to find time for fun and exercise. Get out of bed the same time on weekends as during the week. In addition to freeing up more time for your weekend fitness forays, you'll also regulate your body clock better. Once your body gets used to a regular wake and sleep schedule, you'll fall asleep faster, feel

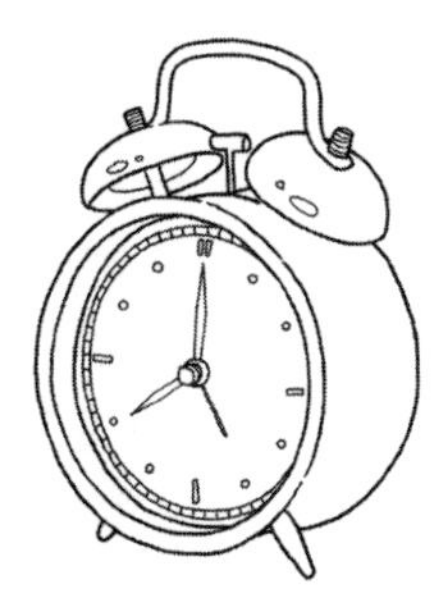

more refreshed when you wake, and avoid that Monday morning "hungover" feeling.

2 **Go for a walk first thing in the morning.** Heading out the door before the Sunday newspaper, rolls, and coffee ensures you fit in your workout. Once you return, you'll feel invigorated and be more likely to stay active during the rest of the day.

3 **Always commit one day to fun.** Never let errands and work spread to both Saturday and Sunday. Whether you live alone or with a family, pick one of those days and go to a water park, take a hike in the mountains, or spend the day playing softball, badminton, or other games in the backyard. You and your companions will soon look forward to this day, devoted not to formal exercise but to fun activities you can do together.

4 **Match your time watching sports with playing sports.** Too many people have become addicted to watching sports on television. For every hour you watch sports on TV, commit to thirty minutes of doing a sport or some other exercise. Gradually increase the ratio to one-to-

one, so an hour watching equals an hour doing. For all the joys of major league sports, nothing compares to hitting a home run, scoring a goal, making a birdie, finishing the race, or winning the tennis match yourself.

5 **Spiff up the yard—manually.** Yard work—leaf raking, garden digging, and mowing—builds upper body strength, burns excess calories, and has been found to be the best physical activity for preventing osteoporosis. Don't make it too convenient for yourself. Physically rake the leaves rather than using a leaf blower; use a push mower rather than a self-propelled one. The more you use your body, the more calories you'll burn, and you can feel good knowing that the less you use gas-powered equipment, the less pollution you've released into the air.

6 **If you cycle, go for a long ride.** During the week you probably can't ride much, but weekends allow you the luxury of riding for half the day or more, if you're so inclined. Scout out a local route

or put the bike in the car and drive to a great riding location. Bring along plenty of food and stash it in your backpack. Take some cash as well, in case you ride past a bagel or coffee shop and want to take a pit stop.

7 **Keep a list of weekend fitness activities and choose one every weekend.** The more varied your fitness routine, the more likely you'll stay active on the weekends. You might enjoy hiking, kayaking, walking, cycling, bird-watching, and other activities.

8 **Keep a fitness kit in your car.** Stock your car with fitness items like a volleyball, soccer ball, baseball and mitts, and a basketball. Make sure to include a pair of sneakers. You never know when you'll find yourself away from home with a little downtime. If your fitness kit is stocked and ready, you'll have everything you need for fun.

9 **Train for a race.** Whether you walk, run, cycle, or do some other sport, signing up for a race will give you the incentive to train on the weekends. Suddenly, fitness becomes the top priority in your life. Serious athletes complete their longer

workout sessions on the weekends, when they have time away from work.

10 **Combine physically active work with pure indulgence.** For instance, split some wood or gather kindling in the woods as the physical activity part of your day, then sit in front of the fire with someone special for the pure indulgence part. Clean up the yard by day and have a barbecue that evening. Take a long hike and have a wonderful picnic basket waiting for you in the car.

11 **Coach or assist your kids' teams.** Instead of spending the weekend with your butt glued to the driver's seat as you shuttle your kids from one activity to another, join them. Sign up to coach their Little League, soccer, or swim team, or help manage things along the sidelines. It'll get you out of the car and you'll exercise all parts of your body—and soul.

12 **Join the kids outside.** Don't just push them out the door and spend the afternoon inside reading or cleaning. Find a tall tree and climb it with them, play a friendly game of hoops in the driveway, spend the day skating, cycling, or playing tag.

Even if our bodies are aging, we all have some childishness inside us still aching to get out.

13 **Take the family camping.** There's nothing like the great outdoors to put your body in a calorie-burning state, or to create memorable times for your kids. After you've pitched your tent, built your campfire, and secured your site, you can look into other activities such as swimming, canoeing, and hiking. Yes, it is worth all the hassle.

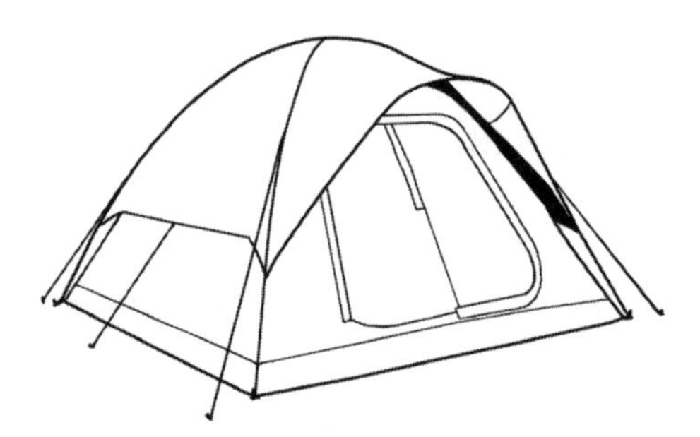

SHARP SENSES

1 **Mix a cup of blueberries with a cup of plain yogurt for breakfast.** Blueberries are one of the richest fruit forms of antioxidants, and a study published in the *Archives of Ophthalmology* found that women and men who ate the greatest amount of fruit were the least likely to develop age-related macular degeneration (ARMD), the leading cause of blindness in older people.

2 **Spread bilberry jam on your morning toast.** Or take a bilberry supplement every morning. Both are readily available online and in some grocery stores. The berries contain compounds called anthocyanosises, which may protect the retina against macular degeneration.

3 **Have spinach twice a week.** Studies find that lutein, a nutrient that is particularly abundant in spinach, may prevent age-related macular degeneration and cataracts. Ideally, get your lutein in combination with some form of fat (such as olive oil) for the best absorption. Make Popeye proud!

4 **Cook with red onions, not yellow.** Red onions contain far more quercetin, an antioxidant that is thought to protect against cataracts. And a little red onion on a salad or sandwich gives a nice extra kick.

5 **Aim your car vents at your feet, not your face.** Dry, air-conditioned air will suck the moisture out of eyes like a sponge. Dry eyes can be more than an inconvenience; serious dryness can lead to corneal abrasions and even blindness if left untreated.

6 **Move your computer screen to just below eye level.** The top line of the screen should be at or below eye level, meaning your eyes should align with the top viewing area of the screen. The screen should be at about twenty-five inches away from your face.

7 **Look away.** Make sure to give your eyes a break by following the 20-20-20 rule. Every twenty minutes take a break; for twenty seconds, look at an object that is twenty feet away. This allows your eyes to relax.

8 **Eat fish twice a week.** A study from Harvard researchers evaluated the diets of 32,470 women and found those who ate the least amount of fish (thus getting the least amount of omega-3 fatty acids) had the highest risk of dry eye syndrome. If you can't eat fish, try fish-oil supplements.

9 **Wear sunglasses.** Make sure they are close-fitting and block 99–100 percent UVA and UVB rays. Wear them anytime you leave the house, even when it isn't sunny outside.

10 **Add a hat.** A wide-brimmed hat or cap will block roughly 50 percent of the UV radiation and reduce the UV radiation that may enter your eyes from above or around your sunglasses.

11 **Roast some fresh beets for an eye-saving side dish.** Beets get their deep red color from phytochemicals called anthocyanins, powerful antioxidants that protect the smaller blood vessels in your body, including those in your eyes.

12 **Replace your mascara every three months and other eye makeup once a year.** Eye makeup is a great repository for bacteria, which can easily be transferred to your eyes and cause infections.

13 **Remove your eye makeup every night before going to bed.** This prevents small pieces of mascara from winding up in your eye and possibly scratching your cornea.

14 **Wear goggles when you're doing carpentry or yard work.** Debris in the eye can lead to corneal abrasions, which can ultimately damage your vision.

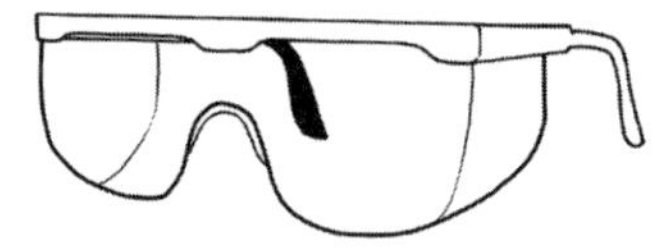

15 **Splurge for extra guacamole!** Guacamole is rich in magnesium. Studies find low levels of magnesium might make you more susceptible to noise-induced hearing loss.

16 **Wear earplugs when doing yard work or at the shooting range.** Any activity that involves loud noises should mean you protect your hearing.

17 **Ask the doctor to clean out the wax in your ears.** Don't try this yourself; sticking pointed objects into your ear canal is a no-no.

18 **Switch to decaf coffee and low-sodium soups.** Caffeine appears to interfere with blood flow to the ear, while salt can lead to fluid retention, which can cause swelling in the functional organs of the ear. Plus, studies found that people with high blood pressure are more likely to have age-related hearing loss than those with normal pressures.

19 **Try a ginkgo biloba supplement.** Some studies suggest the herb might not only help with ringing in the ears, or tinnitus, but may also help treat some types of hearing loss by improving blood flow to the ears. Be patient: the herb takes weeks to work.

20 **Serve food that looks like itself.** Forget fancy-schmancy presentation. If you're serving fish, keep it looking like fish. Your sense of taste is strong if your brain can connect what you're eating with how it looks.

21 **Stay away from the diaper pail and other stinky smells.** Prolonged exposure to bad smells tends to wipe out your ability to smell, says Alan Hirsch, neurological director of the Smell and Taste Treatment and Research Foundation in Chicago. If you must be exposed to such odors on a prolonged basis, wear a mask over your nose and mouth that filters out some of the bad smells.

22 **Add spices to your food.** Even if your sense of smell and taste has plummeted, you should still retain full function in your "irritant" nerve, the nerve that makes you cry when you cut an onion or makes your eyes water when you smell ammonia. So use spices like hot chili powder to spice up your food.

23 **Chew thoroughly and slowly.** This releases more flavor and extends the time that the food lingers in your mouth, so it spends more time in contact with your taste buds. Even before you start chewing, stir your food around. This has the effect of aerating the molecules in the food, releasing more of their scent.

24 **Avoid high-temperature foods and drinks.** They can burn your tongue and damage your taste buds.

25 **Reset your taste for sugar and salt.** Cut them out of your diet for a week. Processed foods have so much sugar and salt that you'll practically stop tasting them if you eat these foods often. Once you switch back, you'll suddenly taste all the salt and sugar you were overlooking.

26 **Try sniff therapy.** It is possible to train your nose (and brain) to notice smells better. Start by sniffing something with a strong odor for a couple of minutes several times a day. Do this continually for three or four months and you should notice your sense of smell getting stronger—at least where that particular item is involved, says Dr. Hirsh.

27 **Clean out your sinuses.** Use a neti pot or a sinus irrigator to clean out your sinuses. It can improve your sense of taste and also help get rid of the bad taste in your mouth that often comes with a sinus infection.

28 **Treat yourself to a comedy festival.** Reward yourself frequently with the gift of laughter. Humor can help you cope better with pain, reduce stress, and even enhance your immune system.

29 **Use it or lose it: the golden rule of brainpower.** Learning new things, varying your routines, having provocative discussions, going on adventurous vacations, and playing a musical instrument all cause your brain to make new connections and function better.

30 **Take a B-complex vitamin pill.** As you age, your body becomes less efficient at absorbing certain B vitamins from food. Yet the Bs are critical for maintaining a sharp memory. They can help break down homocysteine, which in high levels is associated with greater risk of dementia and Alzheimer's disease. The Bs also help produce energy need to develop new brain cells.

31 **Memorize a poem every day.** It may remind you of school, but it is also a great exercise for your memory muscles.

32 **Do one thing every day that will force you out of your comfort zone.** It may be taking a different route to work or writing or using the mouse with your nondominant hand. This kind of challenge is the perfect "weightlifting" exercise for those brain cells.

33 **Listen to music while you are exercising.** A study of thirty-three adults undergoing cardiac rehabilitation found that those who listened to music while they worked out improved their scores on a verbal fluency test—a test that measures overall brainpower.

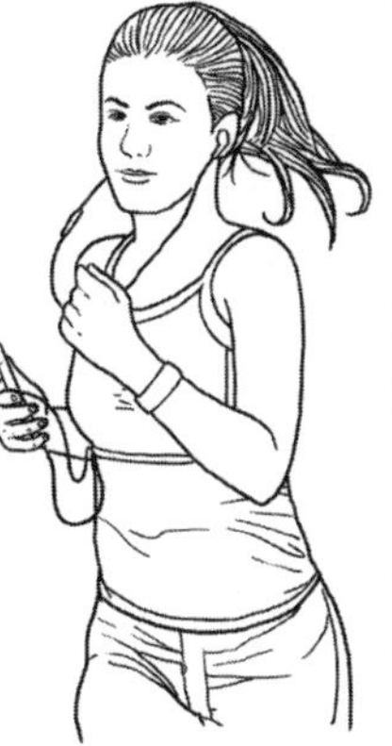

34 **Get a course book from your local college.** Pick one class to take next semester. A study from Chicago's Rush Alzheimer's Disease Center found that people who had higher levels of education exhibited fewer signs of Alzheimer's disease even when autopsies revealed they *had* the disease.

35 **Do one thing at a time.** If you're trying to have a phone conversation while checking email, chances are good you won't remember a word you talked about. A growing body of research finds our increasing tendency to multitask actually harms our brains.

36 **Have a bag of tasty pumpkin seeds.** They are high in iron and shown to improve test scores in college students—making them a perfect brain-boosting snack.

37 **Put tofu cubes into your soup.** Soy products, like tofu, have isoflavones that also appear to help preserve memory and hinder protein changes that contribute to Alzheimer's.

38 **Study, read, and work in a quiet room.** Studies find that noise exposure can slow your ability to rehearse things in your mind, a way of building memory links.

39 **Rekindle your love of reading.** A book, magazine, or newspaper is much more rewarding than watching television. And it's much healthier, because it keeps your brain highly active and engaged. Pick a topic about which you know very little—your brain will soak up the knowledge like a parched rosebush, sending out blooms in the form of neurons that help maintain a healthy memory.

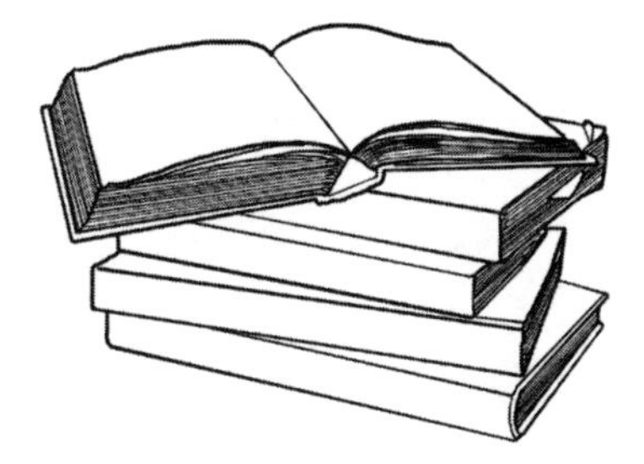

MAINTAINING MENTAL HEALTH

1 **When you're nervous, tighten and release your abdominal muscles over and over again.** You'll strengthen your abs and take your mind off your anxiety. This is a particularly good exercise for when you are nervous about an upcoming speech or presentation.

2 **Fill your office with plants to reduce stress.** By arranging them within eyesight, near your computer, plants significantly lower workplace stress and enhance productivity as well as improving air quality. One suggestion is rosemary; studies find the scent of rosemary to be energizing. Rub one of the sprigs

between your fingers to release the fragrance into the air or clip off a sprig and rub it on your hands, face, and neck to saturate yourself in the scent.

3 **Schedule a mental health day.** It's time for a day off if you're experiencing an unusual number of headaches, neck pain, back pain, other ailments, or find you have trouble falling or staying asleep, or are snapping at your coworkers for no reason. Check your calendar for the upcoming week and pencil in the day you're going to call in sick. This is not lying—you *are* sick, it's just mental rather than physical. Up to 80 percent of visits to primary care physicians are for stress-related complaints.

4 **Write in your journal for ten minutes.** Many people eschew keeping a journal because they can't stand the pressure to write in it every night. But if you limit yourself to just ten minutes, suddenly what seemed like a chore takes less time than washing the dishes. Try listing what you did that day, things that made you smile, things that made you angry—and why they

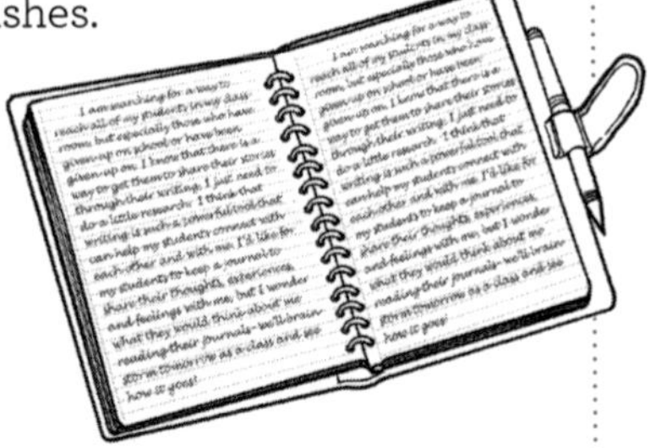

made you angry. Regular journaling is a stress buster, and it's fun to leaf back through your journal and see what you were doing a year before. It provides a way of marking your life in a world in which our lives seem to stream by too fast.

5 **Talk to yourself.** Be kind to yourself. Remind yourself of your strengths, how you handled situations in the past. Be as compassionate with yourself as you would be with a friend.

6 **Break out of your routine today.** Sometimes being stuck in a rut is just that. Get out of it and your mood may come along with you. Take a day off work and go explore a town nearby. Go out to a restaurant for dinner—even though it's a Tuesday night.

7 **Go outside.** Fresh air, sun, and getting your blood moving and endorphins pumping can help with anxiety, depression, and stress.

8 **Call a friend.** Sharing anxieties, fears, stress, and anger with a friend can take the load off your mind and provide some much-needed advice/wisdom. Research shows that production and repair of

brain cells improves through interacting with others.

9 **Sleep.** Our brains require sleep to function properly. Follow the hacks in this book and do what you need to do to get your seven to nine hours every night.

10 **Plan a virtual vacation.** Whether or not you take it doesn't matter. Check out airline costs, pick a hotel, and virtually (but not really) book a snazzy red convertible to drive while you're there. Write down all the details and save any pictures you find, then file them into a vacation journal. Do this once a month, each in a different location and for a different purpose (golf, family, adventure, spa) to provide a pleasant way to unwind before bed.

11 **Write down your entire to-do list for the next day.** In only five minutes, the peace of mind you'll get is priceless. Instead of running a to-do list over and over in your mind—which makes your responsibilities morph into gargantuan proportions—you can enjoy the rest of your evening and have a better shot at falling asleep easily. A reminder app on your phone works well for this purpose.

12 **Write a "done" list.** This is a list of everything you've accomplished today. It's guaranteed to give you a sense of accomplishment and take some stress off your shoulders.

13 **Pour a cup of boiling water over a handful of chamomile leaves.** Or a chamomile tea bag. The herbal mix, long known for its gentle, soothing properties, will help you to de-stress and center yourself.

14 **Drop in on a yoga class.** Just one class is all you need to lower levels of the stress hormone cortisol, according to a study from Jefferson Medical College. Researchers took blood samples

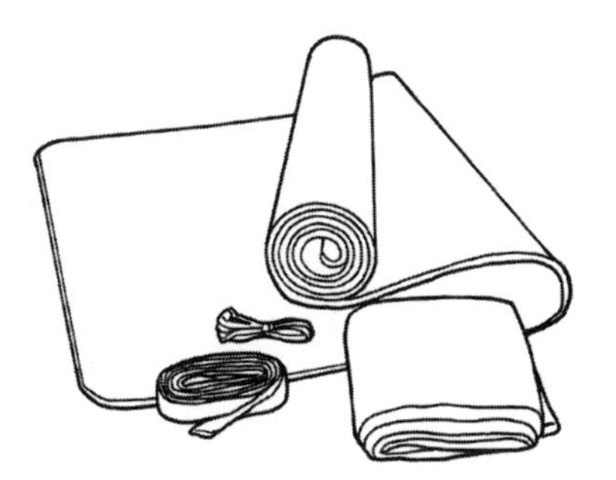

from sixteen beginners taking their first week of yoga classes. Cortisol levels dropped after the first class.

15 **Just say no.** Stress comes from having more demands—emotional, professional, and so on—than you have resources to deal with them. Reduce those demands by delegating responsibilities and duties.

16 **Keep your power.** People will wrong you; life won't go your way. Don't obsess over it and give those things more power over you. It also just wastes time. Use that time doing something healthier and take that power back.

17 **Be nice.** When you are, you'll feel better. Wish someone, anyone, happiness and a relief from their suffering. Sounds corny, but it works.

18 **Learn from your mistakes.** Everyone fails sometimes, but these failures contain the seeds for your next success. Remember that the next time things go south and you'll be happier and healthier for it.

19 **Smile more.** Studies have shown that when people smile even when stressed out, they experience a mood boost. The smile sends a signal to the brain that tell it you're happy and releases endorphins, which reduce stress.

20 **Cherish the moment.** According to the American Psychological Association, focusing on the past can lead to depression, and fearing the future contributes to anxiety. Now is all we have.

21 **Watch your social media intake.** Constantly checking email, Facebook, Twitter, and so on can be a waste of time leading to frazzled nerves and unhealthy comparisons with others.

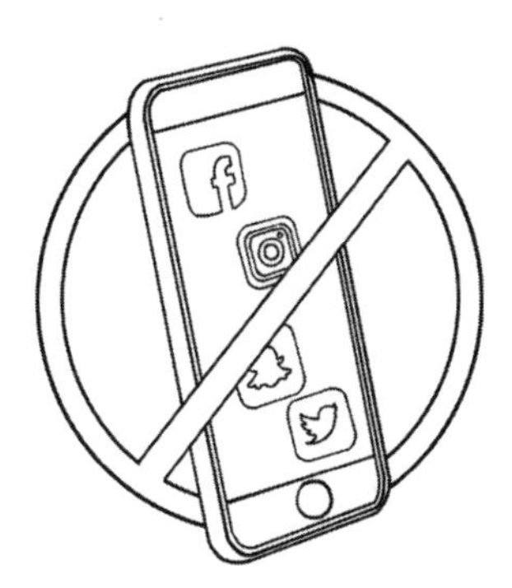

22 **Forgive.** Exacting revenge on someone else only causes long-term grief—and unhealthy consequences—for you.

23 **Stop trying to change others.** Deal with these problem people by accepting them for who they are, detaching from their unacceptable behavior, and defining boundaries.

24 **Get inspired.** Reading inspirational articles and books, even simple quotes, can help you find a new way of thinking about your old problems.

25 **Practice gratitude.** We don't always feel gratitude, but if we practice it our gratitude muscle grows stronger. Take one minute each morning and evening to reflect on what you like or love and what others have done for you throughout your life. Do it daily and share with someone your commitment to doing this.

26 **Volunteer.** Helping others has been shown to reduce stress, anxiety, and anger. Researchers have measured hormones and brain activity that shows being helpful to others brings immense pleasure. The more we give, the happier we feel.

27 **Get help when you need it.** Don't let social stigmas associated with mental health create self-doubt or shame. Don't isolate yourself but seek support from such resources as the National Alliance on Mental Illness (NAMI), which offers free information, support groups, and local programs.

SKIN, HAIR, AND NAILS

1 **Skip the long, steamy showers and opt for shorter, cooler sprays.** Long, hot showers strip skin of its moisture and wash away protective oils. Limit showers to ten minutes and keep the water cool.

2 **Check the dryness of your skin.** If scratching a small area on your arm or leg with your fingernail leaves a white mark, your skin is indeed dry and needs both moisture and exfoliation.

3 **Treat your neck and chest like an extension of your face.** Your neck and upper chest area is covered by very sensitive skin, making it a prime spot for telltale signs of aging such as dryness, sunspots, and wrinkles. To keep this area youthful,

use facial cleansing creams that hydrate and cleanse gently rather than deodorant soaps, which can be drying. Top it all off with a good facial moisturizing cream. If this area is extra dry, use a facial moisturizing mask twice a month.

4 **Humidify your bedroom every night in the winter.** By moisturizing the air in your bedroom, not only will it ease itchy, dry skin, but you'll be able to breathe the moist air more easily.

5 **Switch from a deodorant soap to one with added fat.** These include Dove, Oilatum, or Neutrogena. Deodorant soaps can be drying, whereas added-fat soaps leave your skin feeling soothed and smooth.

6 **Try skipping the soap.** Water by itself does a great job of keeping you clean. And it won't strip away vital oils. Skin is the largest organ in your body, with its own microbiome and protective layer. Soaps can damage this layer and take away the good bacteria along with the bad. Oil cleansers, dry brushing, or your own homemade all-natural scrub all can keep

you clean and your skin healthy. If you must, use a mild cleanser just for the important parts, your armpits and genitals. Try it for a week; your skin will thank you.

7 **Keep your beauty products clean and simple, particularly if you have sensitive skin.** Stay away from products with color, fragrance, or those that produce bubbles or have "antibacterial" on the label. These can all irritate skin.

8 **Use olive oil to refresh and hydrate.** Smooth a couple of drops over your face, elbows, knees, and the backs of your arms every evening. The oil contains monounsaturated fat, which moisturizes without leaving a greasy residue.

9 **Tone your skin with a sage, peppermint, and witch hazel combination.** Sage helps to control oil, peppermint creates a cool tingle, and witch hazel helps restore the skin's protective layer. Combine four ounces of witch hazel with one teaspoon each of sage and peppermint leaves and steep for one to three days before applying to your skin.

10 **Select a moisturizer that contains skin-repairing humectants.** Humectants attract water when applied to your skin and improve its hydration. Good ones include glycerin, propylene glycol, and urea. Also look for skin products that contain alpha-hydroxy acids (AHAs), compounds that help reduce wrinkles and improve dry skin, acne, and age spots. AHAs, which naturally occur in grapes, apples, citrus, and sour milk (think buttermilk or yogurt), work by speeding up the turnover of old skin cells, making skin look younger.

11 **Use a loofah daily to keep ingrown hairs and scaly skin under control.** While in the shower, gently scrub bumpy or scaly skin with a circular motion to remove dead cells. For extra-smooth skin, sprinkle a few drops of an alpha-hydroxy product on the loofah before scrubbing.

12 **Take rose hips every morning to help build collagen.** Rich in vitamin C, rose hips can help keep skin smooth and youthful. Be sure to follow label directions.

13 **Avoid scented lotions and perfumes in the sun.** Scented products can lead to blotchy skin when exposed to the sun.

14 **Apply ice (wrapped in a towel) to dry, itchy skin.** A few minutes on, a few minutes off. Allow the moist cold to relieve your skin and draw warming blood to it, but don't let your skin get so cold as to sting or hurt. An ice pack will work as well!

15 **Smooth aloe vera gel over extra-dry skin.** The acids in aloe eat away dead skin cells and speed up the healing process. Cut off an end of an aloe leaf, split open, and spread the gel on the dry area.

16 **Plunk your rough, dry elbows into grapefruit halves.** First exfoliate your elbows in your bath or shower, then cut a grapefruit in half and rest one elbow on each half, letting them soak for fifteen minutes. The acid in the grapefruit provides extra smoothing power.

17 **Hang room-darkening shades in your bedroom.** They help avoid sleep disturbances or insomnia caused by ambient light. Sleep is critical to your skin's health because most cell repair and regeneration occurs while you're sleeping. If you're not getting enough rest, your skin cannot renew itself.

18 **Cook with garlic every day.** Skin cells grown in a culture dish and treated with garlic had seven times the life span of cells grown in a standard culture. They also tended to look healthier and more youthful than untreated cells. Plus, garlic extract dramatically inhibited the growth of cancerous skin cells.

19 **Do anything that gets you sweating.** Go for a run, ride your bike, or work out in the garden on a hot day. Sweating is nature's way of eliminating toxic chemicals that can build up under skin. Regular exercise maintains healthy circulation and blood flow throughout your body, including your skin. If you're exercising outdoors, though, remember to wear a sunscreen on your face that protects against UVA and UVB rays, or a moisturizer with sunscreen protection.

20 **Grill salmon brushed with olive oil and sprinkled with toasted, crushed walnuts.** There, you've just gotten a skin-healthy dose of poly- and monounsaturated fats, particularly omega-3 fatty acids, which may affect the amount of sun and aging damage your skin experiences. By extension, make sure olive oil is the primary source of fat in your cooking every day, and try to have salmon twice a week or more.

21 **Switch moisturizers every time the seasons change.** Your skin needs more moisture in the winter than in the summer. The same day you bring those sweaters down from the attic for the winter, buy a heavier moisturizer. When you trade in the sweaters for shorts, switch to a lighter one.

22 **Add a teaspoon of grapeseed oil to your toner.** The oil acts as an anti-aging serum by helping your skin cells repair and rejuvenate themselves.

23 **Avoid these three skin destroyers:** Smoking, tanning salons, and sunbathing. All three will age your skin prematurely, many doctors agree.

24 **For double protection, apply a cream containing vitamin C to your face over your sunblock.** The cream helps prevent facial skin damage, dehydration, and wrinkles. Also try creams containing vitamin E or beta-carotene.

25 **Use a spritzer with rose, sandalwood, or bergamot essential oils mixed with water.** These oils are great for hydrating the skin. To create an herbal spritzer, mix a few drops of essential oil with water in a small spray bottle and spritz on your face whenever your skin needs a little boost. Your skin is more pliable when it's hydrated, so a spray helps stave off frown lines and general movement wrinkles, keeps pollutants out and your skin's natural lubricants in. Also, your makeup will stay on longer and look more natural.

26 **Make your own cleansing, moisturizing masks.** Mix one tablespoon plain yogurt with a few dashes of sesame oil and apply. Or mash a banana well and mix with a little honey for an

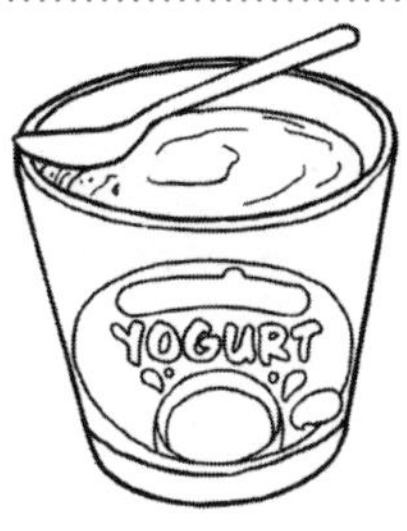

instant dry-skin fix. Or mix a quarter cup whipping cream, half a teaspoon olive oil, two tablespoons ripe mashed avocado, and one teaspoon calendula petals. You can also lightly scramble an egg and apply to your face while still warm, leaving it on until it hardens.

27 **Remove skin-damaging pollutants.** Clean your face and neck with a natural cold cream and follow with a rosewater and glycerin rinse twice a day.

28 **Keep your hands off your face!** Because your hands touch so many surfaces, they are a magnet for dirt and germs. Rub your eyes, stroke your chin, cup your cheek, and you've transferred everything on your hands to your face. As an extension of this, use headphones or a headset when talking on the phone. This, too, keeps hands and germs away from your face.

29 **Stop with one glass of wine or one alcoholic drink.** Overdoing it enlarges the blood vessels near the surface of your facial skin.

30 **De-shine your face throughout the day.** Periodically dab on loose powder to blot excess oil. Don't use pressed powder, which actually contains oil as an ingredient.

31 **Never, ever rub your eyes—apply compresses instead.** The skin on your face is extremely delicate, especially under your eyes. Use a very light touch on your face at all times. If your eyes itch, apply a cold compress or washcloth to the area, or try a cotton pad moistened with toner or witch hazel.

32 **Take one to three 250-milligram capsules of borage oil, evening primrose oil, or flaxseed oil one to three times a day.** All are rich in omega-3 fatty acids like gamma-linolenic acid, great for keeping hair (and nails) moisturized.

33 **Check the drain after each shower for the amount of hair.** The typical person loses from fifty to two hundred hairs a day (out of 80,000 to

120,000 hairs on the head). So it's normal to have a very small clump of hair left on the drain after washing. But if that amount starts increasing, see your doctor. It could mean your scalp has an infection, or that baldness is beginning to set in, or in rarer circumstances, that you have a nutritional deficiency.

34 **Make a shampoo omelet.** Mix one egg with a small amount of shampoo, apply to your hair for five minutes, and rinse well. This helps to feed the protein in your hair.

35 **Bathe your hair in botanical oils.** Available at health food stores, olive, jojoba, and sweet almond oils are all wonderful elixirs for hair. If your hair is thick and heavy, coconut oil works wonders. Dampen your hair and apply small amounts of the botanical oil until your hair is thoroughly covered. Cover with a shower cap and warm towel for a half hour, then rinse and shampoo as usual.

36 **Only spritz three times with hair spray.** In addition to making you look like you just stepped out of 1962, too much hair spray can weigh down your hair, leaving it flat. Instead, try a bionutrient styling spray containing the B vitamin panthenol. It will condition your hair and help protect it from environmental and styling damage.

37 **Protect against split ends.** Wrap wet hair gently in a towel and let the cotton absorb the moisture for a few minutes instead of rubbing.

38 **Keep your hair bouncy and healthy.** Occasionally shampoo your roots only and then apply conditioner to just your ends. Then rinse.

39 **Dry your hair 90 percent only.** To reduce damage to your tresses and add pouf to your do, dry your hair until 90 percent of the moisture is removed, then stop. Most people falsely believe they must use a hair dryer until their hair is bone-dry. Not true. The style should fall into place if your hair is healthy and well cut.

40 **If you usually wear your hair in a ponytail, give it a break.** Take it out for a few hours a day. Also, try not to pull hair back too tightly too often; repeatedly pulling on the hair can lead to traction alopecia.

41 **Protect your hair from harsh pool chemicals.** Comb conditioner through your hair before hitting the pool. When you finish with your swim, rinse with a quarter cup apple cider mixed with three-quarters cup water to help cleanse hair, then follow with more conditioner. Do the same before hitting the beach.

42 **Mash a ripe avocado (pit removed) with one egg, then apply to wet hair.** Avocados are rich in vitamins, essential fatty acids, and minerals that will help restore luster to your hair. Eggs provide protein that helps protect against split ends and heat damage. Leave on for at least twenty minutes, then rinse several times. Repeat once a week for damaged hair and once a month for healthy hair.

43 **Use a gentle shampoo for oily hair.** Ironically, harsh shampoos can actually lead to more oil because your scalp tries to compensate. Use a shampoo that's gentle enough for everyday use.

44 **Join the No Poo movement.** Many health bloggers are ditching their daily shampoo routines and claiming softer, healthier, bouncier hair using just water or a combination of baking soda and apple cider vinegar. Dissolve a tablespoon of baking soda in a cup of water until smooth. Apply the solution to your hair and massage gently and then rinse. Moisturize, if needed, with an apple cider rinse: one part apple cider to two parts water. Voilà. You look mahvelous, darling.

45 **Keep your nails hydrated.** Rub a small amount of petroleum jelly into your cuticle and the skin surrounding your nails every evening before you go to bed or whenever your nails feel dry. Keep a jar in your purse, desk drawer, and car or anywhere you might need it. If you're not a fan of petroleum jelly, substitute castor oil. It's thick and contains vitamin E, which is great for your cuticles, or head to your kitchen cupboard and grab the olive oil, which also works to moisturize your nails.

46 **Wear rubber gloves whenever you do housework.** Most household chores like gardening, scrubbing the bathroom, and washing dishes are murderous on your nails. To protect your digits from dirt and harsh cleaners, cover them with vinyl gloves whenever it's chore time. And for extra hand softness, apply hand cream before you put on the rubber gloves.

Avoid ingrown toenails. Trim your toenails straight across. This is particularly important if you have diabetes. Diabetes affects blood flow to your feet, and any cut, scrape, or ingrown toenail can quickly become infected.

Don't risk a fungal infection. Dry your hands for at least two minutes after doing the dishes, taking a bath/shower, and so on. Also dry your toes thoroughly after swimming or showering.

Air out your work boots and athletic shoes. Better yet, keep two pairs and switch between them so you're never putting your feet into damp, sweaty shoes, which could lead to fungal infections.

50

Wear 100 percent cotton socks. They're best for absorbing dampness, thus preventing fungal infections.

51 **Take biotin to make your nails strong and resilient.** Take 300 micrograms of the B vitamin biotin four to six times a day. Long ago, veterinarians discovered that biotin strengthened horses' hooves, which are made from keratin, the same substance in human nails. Swiss researchers found that people who took 2.5 milligrams of biotin a day for five and a half months had firmer, harder nails. In a U.S. study, 63 percent of people taking biotin for brittle nails experienced an improvement.

52 **Add zinc to your daily diet.** The zinc in just a glass of milk and a hard-boiled egg will do wonders for your nails, especially if your nails are spotted with white, a sign of low zinc intake.

53 **File your nails correctly.** To keep your nails at their strongest, avoid filing in a back-and-forth motion—only go in one direction. And never file

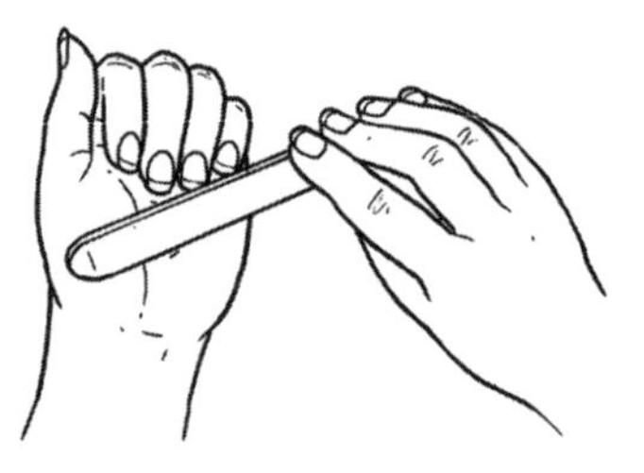

just after you've gotten out of a shower or bath—wet nails break more easily.

54 **Massage your nails to keep them extra strong and shiny.** Nail buffing increases blood supply to the nail, which stimulates the matrix (root tissue) of the nail to grow.

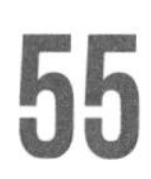

Polish your nails, even if it's just with a clear coat. It protects your nails. If you prefer color, use a base coat, two thin coats of color, and a top coat. Color should last at least seven days but should be removed after ten days.

56 **Avoid polish removers with acetone or formaldehyde.** They're terribly drying to nails. Use acetate-based removers instead.

A BIGGER AND BETTER SMILE

1 **Go on a white-teeth diet.** If you're quaffing red wine, black tea, colas, gravies and dark juices, or smoking cigarettes or cigars, expect the results to show up as not-so-pearly whites. Step one: brush your teeth immediately after eating or drinking foods that stain teeth. Step two: regularly use a good bleaching agent, either over-the-counter or in the dentist's office. Step three: be conscious of the foods and drinks in your diet that can stain your teeth, and eat only when a toothbrush is around, or eat an apple for dessert—it will provide some teeth-cleaning action.

2 **Hum while you brush.** The ideal amount of time to brush in order to get all the bacteria-packed plaque out is at least two minutes. This is why

electric toothbrushes signal every thirty seconds for a total of two minutes. Humming a song works well also.

3 **Grip your toothbrush like a pencil.** Does your toothbrush look like it just cleaned an SUV? If so, you're probably brushing too hard. Contrary to what some scrub-happy people think, brushing with force is not the best way to remove plaque. The best way to brush is by placing your toothbrush at a forty-five-degree angle against your gums and gently moving it in a circular motion, rather than a back-and-forth motion.

4 **Use alcohol-free mouthwash to rinse away bacteria.** Most over-the-counter mouthwashes have too much alcohol, which can dry out the tissues in your mouth, making them more susceptible to bacteria. Some studies even suggest a link between mouthwashes containing alcohol and an increased risk of oral cancer. To be safe, be a teetotaler when it comes to choosing a mouthwash.

5 **Even if you're a grown-up, avoid sugary foods.** Sugar plus bacteria equals oral plaque. Plaque leads to bleeding gums, tooth decay, and cavities. Plus, the acid in refined sugars and carbonated beverages dissolves tooth enamel.

6 **Instead, eat "detergent" foods.** Foods that are firm or crisp help clean teeth as they're eaten. We already mentioned apples (otherwise known as nature's toothbrush); other choices include raw carrots, celery, and popcorn. For best results, make "detergent" foods the final food you eat in your meal if you know you won't be able to brush your teeth right after eating.

7 **Gargle with apple cider vinegar in the morning and then brush as usual.** The vinegar helps remove stains, whiten teeth, and kill bacteria in your mouth and gums.

8 **Practice flossing with your eyes shut.** If you can floss without having to guide your work with a mirror, you can floss in your car, at your desk, while in bed, and before important meetings. In which case, buy several packages of floss and scatter them in your car, your desk, your purse, your briefcase, your nightstand.

9 **Check the freshness of your breath.** Lick your palm and smell it while it's still wet. If you smell something, it's time for a sugar-free breath mint.

10 **Suck—don't chew—extremely hard foodstuffs such as peanut brittle, hard candy, or ice.** Chewing these hard foods creates tiny fractures in the enamel of your teeth that, over the years, combine to result in major cracks.

11 **Chuck your toothbrush, or toothbrush head, every two to three months.** Otherwise, you're just transferring bacteria to your mouth.

LOOKING (AND SMELLING) YOUR BEST

1 **Buy clothes made from natural fibers like cotton.** They allow skin to breathe, reducing body odor. Avoid synthetic fibers, such as nylon or spandex, which tend to limit ventilation.

2 **Allow perspiration to evaporate.** Wear loose-fitting clothes to allow air to circulate around your body. Tight-fitting clothes cause sweat to be trapped in a film on your skin, which can result in body odor or noticeable perspiration stains.

3 **Apply antiperspirant at the right time.** When your underarms are a little moist, like right after a warm shower or bath, apply your antiperspirant. It enables active ingredients to enter the sweat glands more readily.

4 **Try a sink bath.** When time is short, but you need to be at your freshest, fill your sink with water and add four tablespoons baking soda. Then dip a sponge or washcloth in the sink and rub yourself down.

5 **Avoiding ingrown hairs.** Lather with shaving cream or gel for five minutes to soften hairs. Then shave in the direction of the hair growth with a new blade. Follow with a gentle moisturizer.

6 **Shave slow and short.** Your skin is not flat, so long strokes increase your chances of cuts or

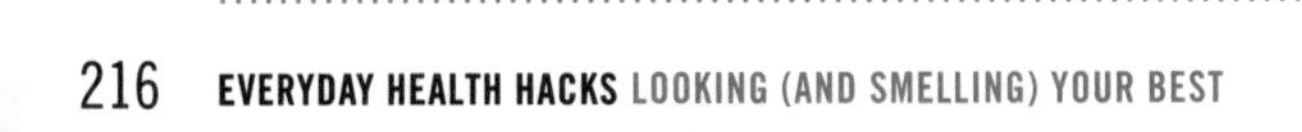

scrapes. Use short strokes and rinse the blade often in hot water. Go slowly and try not to press down with the blade, especially around sensitive areas.

7 **Apply your shaving cream with a shaving brush.** This will give you an extra luscious shaving session (whether for your legs or your face). It will create tons of lather, which will make the hairs softer and easier to remove.

8 **Ward off smelly feet with odor-absorbing insoles.** Foot odor is a very common problem. Keep your feet smelling fresh by scrubbing them daily and drying them completely when you get out of the shower. Then insert into your shoes odor-absorbing insoles, such as Odor-Eaters or a charcoal insert, like Sof Sol or Bamboo Charcoal. Antifungal shoe sprays can also reduce odors.

9 **Keep your shoes smelling sweet.** Try any number of do-it-at-home ideas: put a tea bag in each shoe when you take it off, put a dryer sheet in overnight, or insert a coffee filter and add some baking powder.

10

Apply a cornstarch-based body powder. Do this in the morning to help skin stay drier throughout the day and reduce odor.

11

Reduce odor-causing bacteria. Do this by wiping a cotton ball soaked in rubbing alcohol, vinegar, or hydrogen peroxide onto your underarms during the day. Or try witch hazel or tea tree oil, both of which help keep you dry, kill bacteria, and deodorize.

12

Control foot odor. Use a roll-on antiperspirant across the bottom of your feet, before putting on your socks, to reduce foot odor.

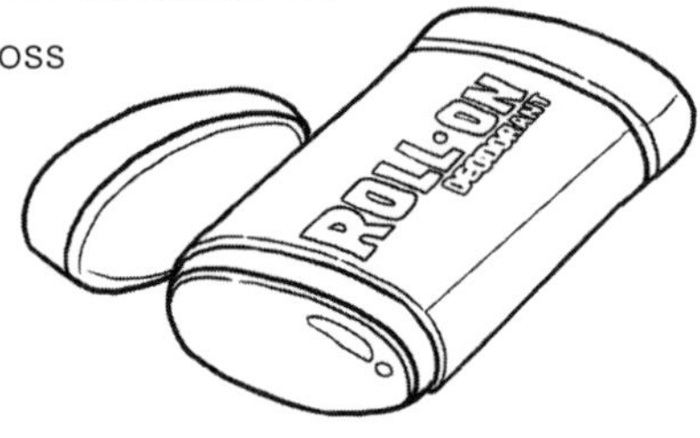

13

Give your daily moisturizer time to penetrate. If your moisturizer doesn't have time to penetrate your skin, your makeup may smear or go on unevenly. Just wait a few minutes before starting to apply your makeup.

14 **Shave after your shower or in the shower!** Steam and hot water soften the bristles of your beard and open up the pores of your skin, making shaving easier and less painful. Most men can get a terrific shave without any lather or cream whatsoever by shaving as the last part of a shower. Five minutes of hot, steamy water provides all the moisture and hair softening your beard needs, and the rinse-off and cleanup take just seconds.

15 **When the weather gets warmer, trim your armpit hair.** There will be less hair to trap bacteria and hence, less odor.

CLEANING HOUSE

1

Clean the things you'd never think to clean. Your mattress is a magnet for allergy-causing dust mites. Washing the mattress cover in very hot water (140°F or more) every month and wiping down the top of the mattress with hot water can go a long way toward reducing morning stuffiness. Other neglected areas include telephones, indoor garbage cans, shower curtains, automatic dishwashers, fireplace, and HVAC filters.

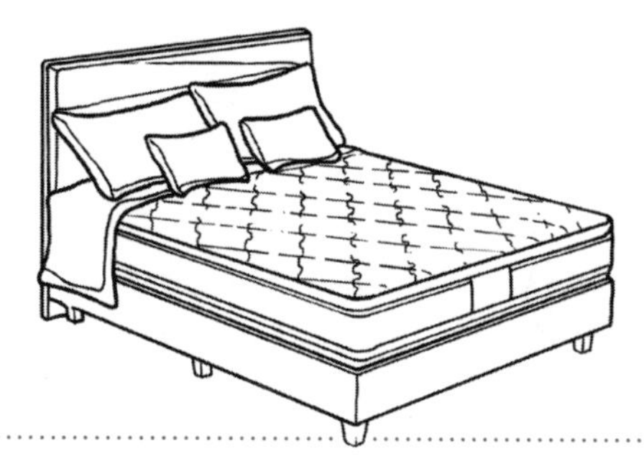

2 **Open your drains the nontoxic way.** Chemical drain cleaners are extremely corrosive and dangerous, containing such toxic ingredients as lye or sulfuric acid. Even the vapors are harmful. Instead, pour a pot of boiling water or toss a handful of baking soda followed by a half cup vinegar down the drain weekly. Also effective in preventing clogs are many brands of enzymatic cleaners, such as Nature's Miracle (used to clean up pet "accidents"), found in pet stores, which use live enzymes that "eat" the bacterial matter that clings to the drains.

3 **Clean your windows the healthy way.** Add one-third cup distilled white vinegar and a spoonful of dishwasher detergent, or a quarter cup rubbing alcohol, to a quart of distilled water. If you're using the latter recipe and your windows streak, don't blame the cleaner. You've probably got a wax buildup from the commercial products you were using before. Switch to the vinegar and dishwasher detergent formula.

4 **Sanitize your toilet bowl safely.** Fill a spray bottle with straight white vinegar and pour a capful of vinegar into the toilet, then spray the

sides of the bowl. Also, sprinkle baking soda in the toilet, wait fifteen minutes, and scrub with a bit of baking soda sprinkled on the brush. Pour one cup of vinegar into the toilet and leave overnight once a month and when you leave for vacation; the vinegar dissolves any alkali buildup to prevent hard-water rings in the toilet. To disinfect the toilet completely, wipe all surfaces with a cloth soaked in rubbing alcohol or with some of the alcohol-based hand cleaner available in stores.

5 Clean out your washing machine and dryer.

High levels of coliform bacteria, an indicator of unsanitary conditions, and diarrhea-causing Escherichia coli have been cultured from home washing machines. When researchers washed sterile clothes in non-bleach laundry detergent, they found that 40 percent emerged contaminated with E. coli bacteria—with enough extra to contaminate the next load. The greatest risk comes when transferring wet laundry with your bare hands to the dryer. Try using rubber gloves when doing your wash and add a cupful of hydrogen peroxide to your loads instead of bleach, and use the hottest water setting.

6 **Disinfect your cutting board.** There can be up to two hundred times more fecal bacteria on the average cutting board in the home than on the toilet seat. To get it clean, run it through the dishwasher, spray it with straight 5 percent vinegar and let it set overnight, or microwave it on high for thirty seconds.

7 **Microwave your kitchen sponges for thirty seconds every day.** The common household sponge may contain 320 million opportunistic bacterial pathogens, enough of which could be transferred from the sponge to your hand to your eyes or mouth to make you sick.

8 **Make your own disinfectant.** Keep a box of borax around because it is a natural product made of sodium, boron, oxygen, and water and is unbeatable for tough cleaning jobs, as a bleach substitute, or mixed with water for a disinfectant.

Rubbing alcohol is another good natural disinfectant. Just don't light any matches around it.

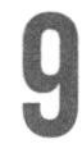

Scrub the floors on your hands and knees once a week. Not only will you have cleaner floors than a mop provides, but you'll also strengthen your arms at the same time.

BEATING BAD HABITS

1 **Make an honest list about your habit.** Make a like/dislike list of your habit. Get feedback from your friends and family. When the negative side outweighs the positive side, you are ready to quit.

2 **Make a list of why quitting won't be easy.** Next to each entry, list one or more options for overcoming that challenge. Examples could be substituting your habit with a healthier habit, creating a support group for yourself, or using visualization techniques to quit.

3 **Set a quit date.** And write a "quit date contract" that includes your signature and that of a supportive witness.

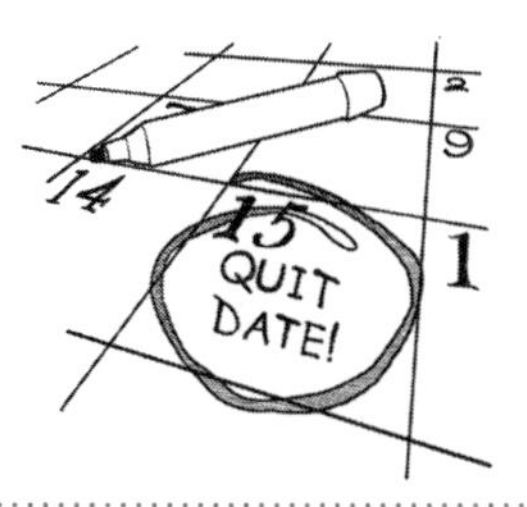

4 **Instead of a cigarette break at work, take a walk.** Or play a game of solitaire or eat a piece of fruit.

5 **Put all the money you're saving on your habit in a large glass jar.** You want to physically see how much you've been spending. Earmark that money for something you've always dreamed of doing but never thought you could afford.

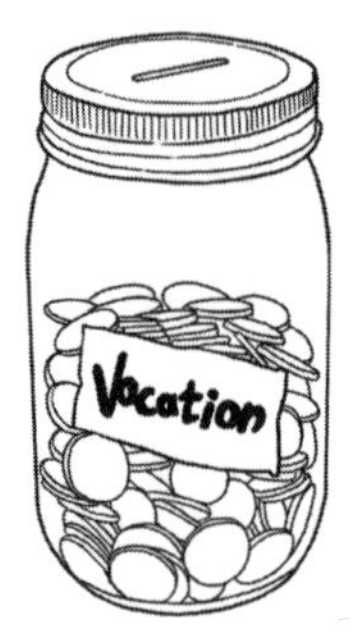

6 **If you relapse, just start again.** You haven't failed. Some people have to quit as many as eight or ten times before they are successful. Take a look at what caused your relapse so you can be prepared for next time.

7 **Meet friends, dates, or business associates at the park or cafe, not a bar.** If the point of the get-together is a fun, casual conversation in a friendly, loose environment, there are many ways to do that without the alcohol.

8 **Switch to mixed drinks with a lower-proof alcohol.** There are lots of alternatives to the standard, high-power alcohol of gin, vodka, or whiskey. For example, a flavored cognac with seltzer has half the alcohol content of a gin drink, and probably twice the flavor.

9 **Keep a habit diary.** Track how often you are partaking in the habit you are trying to reduce/break. Having the visual of how often you do this habit will help you cut down or quit.

10 **Give yourself downtime.** If you are glued to your social media apps, try deleting them for a short period of time, say for the weekend. You can always reinstall them.

11 **Set parental controls.** Most phones have parental controls to help parents limit screen time for their children. Use them on yourself! Sure, you will be able to turn them off, but the extra steps of disabling them might be just enough for you to put down the phone/tablet for the time being.

IN CASE OF EMERGENCY

1. **Keep your first-aid kit stocked.** Besides Band-Aids and painkillers, keep a thermometer handy. This will help you monitor early symptoms of illness.

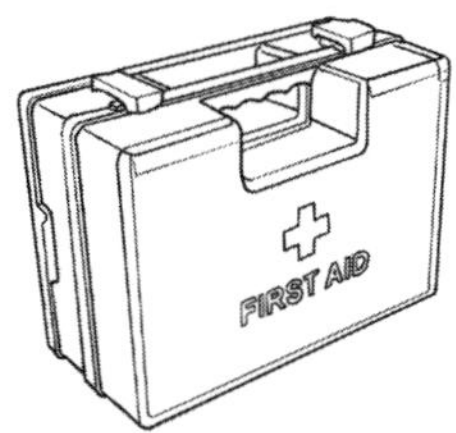

2. **Be informed.** During statewide emergencies, many states and cities will text important information to residents. Make sure to sign up for those emergency texts and/or follow your local government on social media. Keeping up to date on what is happening in your city will help keep you physically safe. New health guidelines may be introduced, and it is important to know what is

happening around you. FEMA has an app you can download for free.

3 **Paperwork.** Nobody wants to be scrabbling around to find important paperwork during an emergency. Keep originals in a safe place (a safe-deposit box or a fire/water safe storage) and have copies with your first-aid kit or scanned and saved in a secure, online location. Knowing where your records are during an emergency will be one less thing for you to worry about. Also, if you have to seek medical help or leave your home, you will have the documents readily available.

4 **Keep in touch.** If you find yourself under quarantine or shelter-in-place orders, it is important to keep in touch with your loved ones. Plan a weekly video chat with you friends. Call your grandparents! During an emergency, it is critical to monitor your mental health as well as your physical health. Keeping in touch with loved ones can help you from feeling isolated or even ease your worries about your family. Checking in on friends and family has benefits for both parties.

5 **Practice good health habits.** Make sure you follow any new health guidelines, and keep up with the classics: wash your hands for at least twenty seconds, stop touching your face, get plenty of sleep, find a way to manage your stress, and find new ways of keeping active.

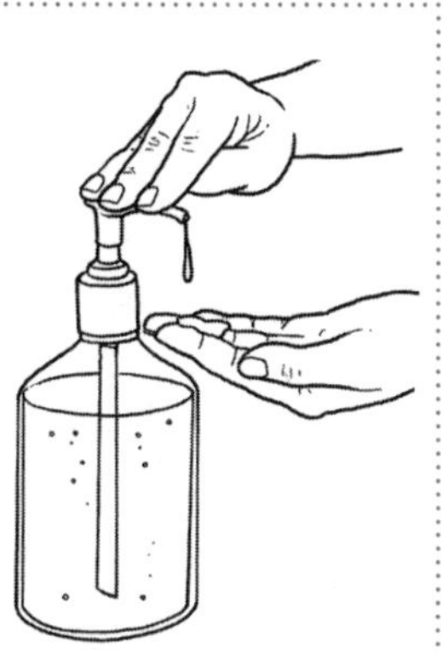

6 **Organize and protect prescription medications to prepare for flooding.** Place medication bottles or packages in a waterproof container or bag, such as a freezer-safe, resealable plastic bag.

7 **Stay up to date.** Know when you're due for a vaccine booster, such as tetanus and seasonal flu.

8 **Know the shelf lives and proper storage temperatures for your prescriptions, including insulin.** Medicines kept in areas with high humidity or fluctuating temperatures, such as a bathroom cabinet, or left in direct light degrade faster and can lose effectiveness.

9 **Talk to your doctor.** People living with diabetes may need to use a different insulin brand or type if their care plan is disrupted. You should work with your doctor if you need to switch insulin. Make sure to closely monitor your blood glucose and seek medical attention as soon as possible.

10 **Mail-order drugs.** Consider signing up for mail-order medication delivery if available. This will come in handy if you are unable to go to the pharmacy due to illness or injury. During a shelter-in-place order due to a flu or other outbreak, it is likely that the mail and delivery will continue.

11 **Replace batteries.** Check the batteries in your carbon monoxide (CO) detectors at least once a month to prevent CO poisoning. CO is an odorless, colorless, and tasteless gas that can cause sudden illness and death if inhaled.

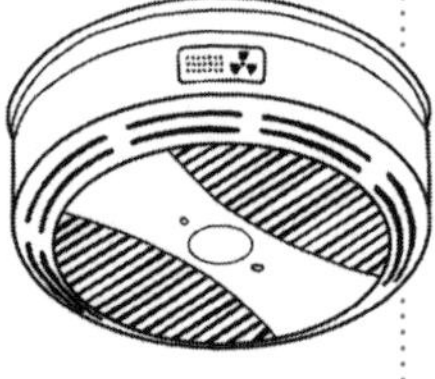

12 **Know where to go.** Pre-identify emergency departments, urgent care centers, dialysis centers, hemophilia treatment centers, veterinarians, and so on near your home and along your designated evacuation route.

13 **Stock up.** If possible, keep a stock of nonperishable and ready-to-eat food, including specialty foods—such as nutrition drinks and ready-to-feed formula—for infants, people with dietary restrictions, food allergies and sensitivities, and medical conditions such as diabetes. To stock up, take advantage of buy-one, get-one-free sales when you are doing your normal shopping. Have at least a three-day supply of nonperishable food for each member of the household. Visit ready.gov for suggestions.

14 **Pack emergency supplies in a portable and durable container(s).** This may include a plastic bin, duffel bag, backpack, trash can with a lid, and/or carry-on luggage.

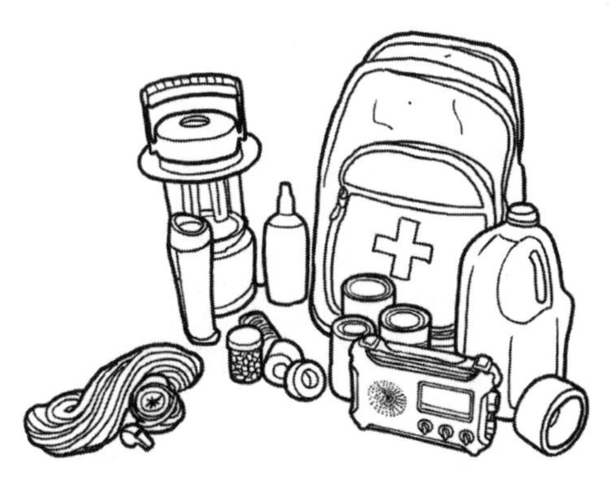

15 **Update your supplies every six months.** Or as the needs of your family change. Remove, use, and replace any food and water, prescription medications, and supplies before they expire.

16 **Store a bottle of unscented liquid household chlorine bleach.** This can be used to disinfect your water and for general cleaning and sanitizing. You can disinfect drinking water by adding two drops of bleach per quart or liter and stirring well (wait a half hour before drinking). Try to store bleach in an area where the average temperature stays around 70°F (21°C). Because the amount of active chlorine in bleach decreases over time due to normal decay, consider replacing the bottle each year.

17 **Have multiple routes.** In the case of an emergency, it is one less thing to stress about if you already have a few different routes or ways of getting home from work.

18 **Determine water needs.** After a natural disaster, clean drinking water may not be available. Experts suggest at least one gallon of water per person per day for three days. The brand

Blue Can Water has a shelf life of fifty years, so consider buying a case or two.

19 **Consider a survival kit.** You may be on your own for days after a natural disaster. Make a kit for your home and car, which includes food (high-energy food bars or freeze-dried food), water, and medical supplies. Several companies sell premade kits, but you can make one yourself for less.

20 **Keep energized.** Have a plan for recharging your phone and other devices. This could be a backup battery or a solar charger.

21 **Don't forget Fido.** He's a member of the family, too, and will be just as affected by an emergency as you are. Make a kit for him too.

22 **Make a plan.** Know what you'll do ahead of time to take care of all family and pets. Where will you shelter? What's your evacuation route? How will you communicate with your family? Ready.gov or redcross.org are both great resources.

KNOW THYSELF

1 **Every evening, think PERF.** Essentially, there are four things you should monitor every day to make sure you are living healthy: the amount of vegetables and fruits you ate that day (produce); whether you walked and were active (exercise); whether you got at least fifteen minutes of laughter and fun time for yourself (relaxation); and whether you got enough beans, grains, and other high-fiber food in your diet (fiber).

2 **Check your hairbrush.** If your hair is falling out, ask your doctor to check your levels of blood ferritin, an indication of how much iron your body is storing. Some studies suggest that low levels may be related to unexplained hair loss. Thyroid disease is another fairly common cause.

3 **Keep a mental color chart of the color of your urine.** Sure it sounds gross, but at least you don't have to pee into a cup to do it. Your urine should be a clear, straw color. If it's dark or has a strong smell you may not be getting enough fluids. If it continues to be dark colored even after you increase your liquid intake, follow up with your doctor. Bright yellow urine? Chalk it up to the B vitamins in your multivitamin.

4 **Check your heart rate after exercise.** Women who had poor heart rate recovery, or HRR, after exercise had twice the ten-year risk of having a heart attack as those who had normal HRR. To test your HRR after regular strenuous activity, count your heartbeats for fifteen seconds, then multiply by four to get your heart rate. Then sit down and wait two minutes before checking again,

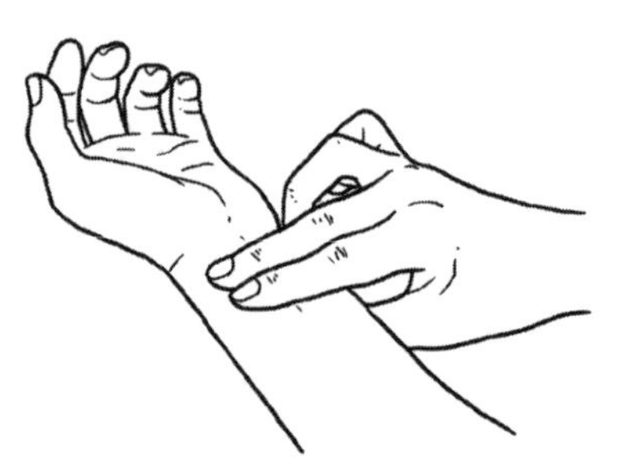

and subtract the second number from the first. If it's under fifty-five, then your HRR is higher than normal and you should follow up with your doctor.

5 **Measure your height every year after you turn fifty.** This is especially important for women as a way of assessing posture and skeletal health. A change in stature can be as informative as a change on a bone density test in terms of assessing your overall bone health. Don't skip the bone density test, though, because it picks up bone loss before your height changes.

6 **If you have diabetes, check your feet every day.** Examine your feet carefully for any blisters, fungus, peeling skin, cuts, or bruises. People with diabetes often have some nerve damage in their extremities, so these daily self-examinations can be critical clues to how well you're monitoring your blood sugar and if you might have nerve damage.

7 **Take a look at yourself.** For men: check for any swelling on the scrotal skin. Examine each testicle with both hands; place the index and middle fingers under the testicle with the thumbs placed

on top, roll the testicle gently between the thumbs and fingers—you shouldn't feel any pain when doing the exam. Don't be alarmed if one testicle seems *slightly* larger than the other. If you find a lump on your testicle, see a doctor, preferably a urologist, right away. For women: using clean hands and the help of a mirror, examine the various parts of the vulva. Take note of the color and size; that way if anything changes you will notice.

8 **Take the fall test.** Time yourself standing on one leg, in shoes or barefoot, but don't hold on to anything. Try it on both legs (one at a time) three times. Aim for at least holding your balance for twelve seconds. If your best leg time is less than that, or you wobble back and forth, you have poor balance and should talk to your doctor or physical therapist about exercises to improve it, because a fall can lead to serious complications if you have osteoporosis.

9 **Check your blood pressure every six months.** You can do this with a home blood pressure cuff, at the drugstore, or at a health fair or screening. If the top number is over 120 and the

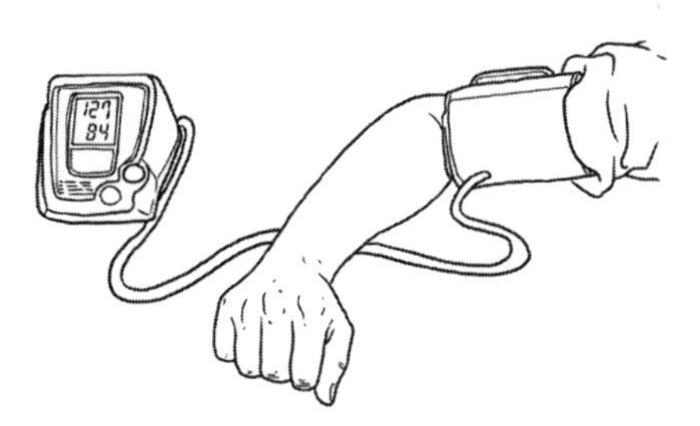

bottom number is higher than 80, wait a day, then check it again. If it's still high, follow up with your doctor.

10 **Check your cholesterol once a year.** This can be done with a home testing kit available at most drugstores, or at a health fair or screening. If your total cholesterol is over 200 mg/dl, follow up with your doctor.

11 **Check the pulse in your feet once every three to six months.** To monitor the circulation in your legs, there are two pulses you should be able to find: one near the middle of the top of your foot (called the dorsalis pedis), and the other right behind the big bony lump on the inside of your ankle (called the posterior tibialis). The posterior tibialis is more important because it's more consistently in the same place. If the pulses become weak or hard to find, follow up with your doctor, especially if you have any leg pain when walking.

12 **Get naked every two to three months.** With a significant other (or *very* close friend) conduct a head-to-toe skin exam looking for any new moles, changed moles, suspicious spots, or rashes. Make sure to check your scalp, between your toes and fingers, and even on the underside of your arms. If you find anything worrisome, follow up with a dermatologist. Do the ABCD test when checking moles: asymmetry—the two halves don't match; border irregularity—the edges are jagged; color—it's not uniform; diameter—it's more than one-quarter inch wide.

13 **Examine your toenails once a month.** Look for early signs of fungal infection or ingrown toenails. Both are best treated early.

14 **Conduct a breast self-exam every month just after your period or on the first of the month.** The American Cancer Society online provides how-to instructions. Also, YouTube has instructional videos. Talk to your doctor about the best time of the month to do your check.

15 **Know your body mass index, or BMI.** This measure has become particularly popular to gauge the health of your weight, because it relates weight to height. A normal BMI is 18.5 to 24.9, a BMI of 25 to 30 puts you in the overweight category, increasing your risk for numerous diseases and health conditions. A BMI above 30 means you are obese, a formal medical condition recognized by the federal government and most insurers. The formula for BMI is weight in kilograms divided by height in meters squared.

16 **Ask your partner if you snore.** Or if you live alone, try recording yourself at night. Harvard researchers found that women who snored were more than twice as likely as those who didn't to develop diabetes—regardless of weight, smoking history, or family history of diabetes. Snoring can also be a sign of sleep apnea; the condition, in which you stop breathing dozens or even hundreds of times during the night, can damage your lungs nearly as much as smoking.

17 **List your pills.** Every time you see your doctor, have a list of the pills you are currently taking, as well as their dosages. This includes prescription medicine, vitamins, herbs, supplements, and over-the-counter drugs. Your doctor will be able to see if there are any problematic combinations or redundancies.

18 **Add a pulse oximeter to your first-aid kit.** It can be important to know your heart rate and oxygen levels. Is your shortness of breath due to a panic attack or something more serious? A pulse oximeter is a small device that estimates how much oxygen is in your blood; most also read your heart rate. These can be found online and in most pharmacies. Prices start around $20.

INDEX